THE HEALING OF 7 CHAKRAS FOR A BALANCED LIFE

A GUIDE TO THE IMPACT OF THE CHAKRAS IN OUR LIFE

PRITMA JASHNANI

Copyright © Pritma Jashnani
All Rights Reserved.

This book has been published with all efforts taken to make the material error-free after the consent of the author. However, the author and the publisher do not assume and hereby disclaim any liability to any party for any loss, damage, or disruption caused by errors or omissions, whether such errors or omissions result from negligence, accident, or any other cause.

While every effort has been made to avoid any mistake or omission, this publication is being sold on the condition and understanding that neither the author nor the publishers or printers would be liable in any manner to any person by reason of any mistake or omission in this publication or for any action taken or omitted to be taken or advice rendered or accepted on the basis of this work. For any defect in printing or binding the publishers will be liable only to replace the defective copy by another copy of this work then available.

Dedicated to the people who want to know about the chakras and how to balance them to lead a balanced life.

Contents

Preface

Every human being has within himself energy centers or chakras which are related to the proper functioning of various organs. They also help us to deeply connect with ourselves and have a deep understanding of life. If any of the chakras become misbalanced, then it can greatly affect us physically, emotionally and psychologically.

I have explained in each chapter the location, color, the element and the seed mantra of each chakra.

Besides this, I have also given the benefits of each chakra when balanced and when it is misbalanced, then what Yoga poses or affirmations to be practiced, to bring it to a balanced position.

At the end I have added an additional chapter to let you know the correct position of each chakra with the help of your fingers, especially little finger and thumb.

Meditation is the best way to visualize the chakra we want to balance and imagining that chakra as a ball of energy which keeps on rotating at its position and radiating energy to all other parts of the body.

To activate the crown chakra or Sahasrara chakra, it is necessary to first activate all the lower chakras. Start right from the root chakra or muladhara, then the Swadishthana, then solar plexus, heart chakra, throat chakra, then Ajna chakra. After all these chakras are active, then only you can easily focus on activating the crown chakra which causes spiritual awakening in you.

Acknowledgements

I express my sincere gratitude to my late mother, late brother, my father and my sisters, without whom it was not possible to express my thoughts in the form of words written in this book.

Though my mother is not with us, but her blessings and love always remains with us. She had a belief that one day I will be writing books and become an author.

I also express my gratitude to the Almighty, whose grace and blessings have helped me to write this book.

About The Author

Pritma Jashnani is the head of the **Centre of Computer Technology,** Lucknow, who has taught several students so far in her career of 25 years.

She has taught more than 3000 students who are now successfully placed in top companies. She has a unique style of teaching. She believes in quality education rather than increasing the number of students.

She has been teaching courses like

Java, Website Designing, Data Structures, Python, Android, and a lot more to B.Tech, MCA, and BCA students.

13 years back, she started writing books for her students so that they do not find any difficulty in the topics they are taught.

She took a lot of time doing research and picking questions from the exam papers of various schools and compiling them into set of two both for class 10th and 12th.

Study Material and Exercise book.

She has also written books on **ASP.NET, PHP, PYTHON, Core Java, C#, Advanced Java, Oracle, etc.**

This is her second book on non-fiction series based on the healing of 7 chakras for healthy living.

She is now writing another book, which will be released soon.

Hope you like this book as it will encourage her to write more books for you.

For Joining any courses, you can contact her by sending mail on jashpritma@gmail.com

You can even buy any study materials on **Java, ANDROID, ASP.NET, C, C++, C#, PHP etc.**

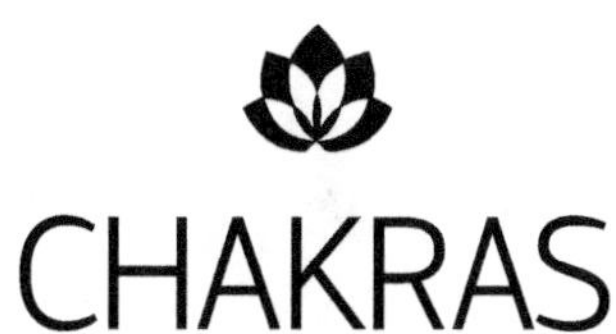

CHAPTER ONE

CHAKRAS

In Sanskrit, Chakra means "disc" or "wheel". There are various energy centers in our body which are referred to as chakras. Various organs of our body are related to these wheels or spinning energy centers.

It is necessary that all the Chakras are balanced so that we are happy, focused, and emotionally strong. The moment any Chakra is imbalanced or blocked, we experience physical or emotional symptoms.

According to Lord Shiva, we have 114 chakras in our body, out of which 7 are major chakras and they are meant to balance the proper functioning of our body and also help us lead a balanced, happy and focused life. These Chakras run through the entire length of the spinal cord, starting from the base or the root and extending upwards to the tip of the head or the crown chakra.

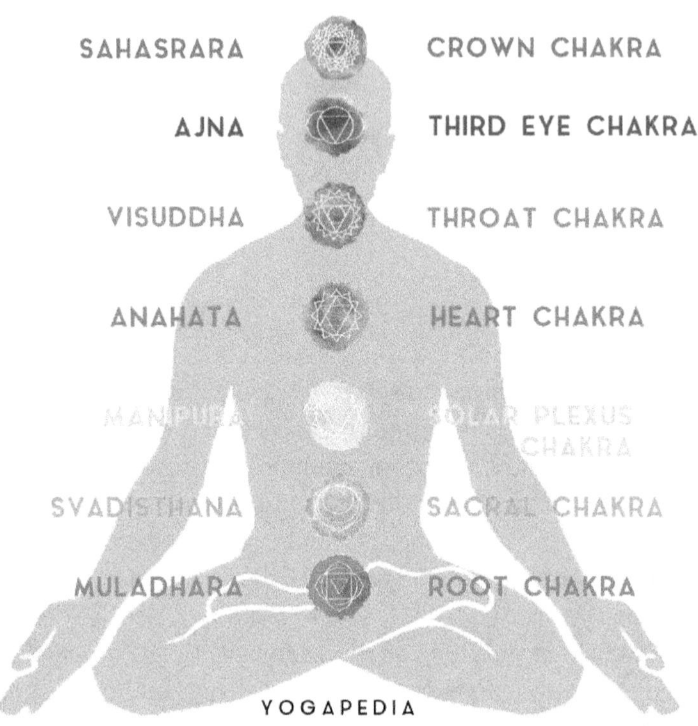

7 chakras

Let us see in brief these Chakras

Root Chakra

This is also known as Muladhara Chakra, located at the base of the spine. It helps us feel grounded to the earth, gives foundation of life and helps us withstand challenges of life. We get a feeling of security.

This Chakra is Red in Color.

Sacral Chakra

The other name of this chakra is Swadishthana chakra. It is present just below the belly button. It is responsible for sexual and creative energy.

If this chakra is balanced, we feel emotionally connected to others and a sense of creativity emerges.

This Chakra is Orange in Color.

Solar Plexus

This is also known as Manipura and is located in the stomach area. This Chakra when active, gives a feeling of self esteem and self-confidence. It helps us control our life and feel confident.

This Chakra is Yellow in Color.

Heart Chakra

This is also known as Anahata Chakra. It is located in the heart region, at the center of the chest. It is related to the feelings of love and compassion and the person is loving in nature.

This Chakra is Green in Color.

Throat Chakra

This is also known as Vishuddhi Chakra. It is located in the throat region and is responsible for verbal communication. The person feels confident while speaking and can express his thoughts with clarity before others.

This Chakra is Blue in Color.

Third Eye Chakra

The other name of this Chakra is Ajna Chakra. It is present in the centre of the forehead between the two eyebrows. It is related to light and provides deep insight and wisdom. It is the center of intuition.

This Chakra is Indigo in Color.

Crown Chakra

The other name of this Chakra is Sahasrara. This is at the top of the head. It represents spiritual connection of us with the divine. It helps us understand our true self and we feel complete in ourselves. This Chakra is violet in color.

Summary

1. There are basically 7 chakras out of 114 Chakras that are essential for proper functioning of our body and keeping us mentally and emotionally balanced.

2. Root Chakra is at the base of spine and is red in color and helps us withstand any challenges of our life.

3. Sacral Chakra is just below the belly button and is related to creativity and emotional connect.

4. Solar Plexus is in the stomach area and gives feeling of self-confidence and helps take control of our life.

5. Heart Chakra is present in the centre of chest, in the heart region. It is related to love and compassion.

6. Throat Chakra is present in the throat region and is responsible for verbal communication.

7. The Third Eye Chakra is related to Intuition and Imagination. It is located between the eyebrows.

8. The Crown Chakra is present at the top of the head and is related to spiritual connectivity of a human being with God.

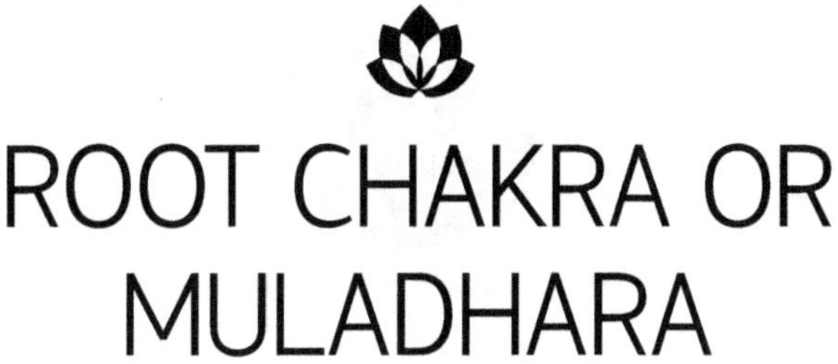

CHAPTER TWO

ROOT CHAKRA OR MULADHARA

Muladhara or the root chakra is situated at the base of the spine. It is red in color and is related to the earth element. This chakra helps us dig deep inside ourselves and feel firmly rooted. It gives us the strength to withstand the challenges of our lives. It helps us feel secure and gives a sense of stability.

Location	Base of spine
Color	Red
Element	Earth
Emotion	Strength to withstand any challenges
Seed Mantra	LAM

Muladhara details

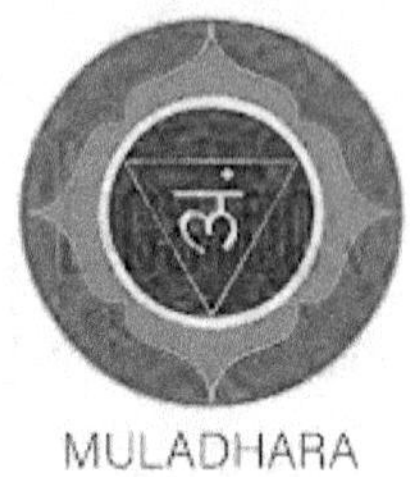

Root Chakra

With a balanced root Chakra, we feel deeply connected to ourselves and to the world. We remain calm and stable at various situations of life and feel deeply grounded to the world.

If the root chakra is misbalanced or blocked then we can experience the following symptoms.

- Anxiety and depression.
- Rushing from one task to another.
- We feel distracted.
- Inability to take action
- Lower back problem.
- Inflammation
- We develop Suicidal thoughts.
- Pelvic pain.
- Colon issues.
- Bladder issues.
- Constipation.
- Weight gain.
- Weight loss.
- Rage(anger)
- Feeling of Insecurity.
- Left arm, legs or foot issues.
- Low self-esteem

Due to Imbalances in this Chakra, we no longer feel a sense of belonging to this world and lose interest.

Some Mental signs are

1. Pessimism
2. Poor focus
3. Negative Outlook.

Eating disorders are

1. Anorexia Nervosa (an eating disorder reflected by an unusual low body weight).

1. Bulimia Nervosa (a serious *eating disorder*, you eat large amounts of food and then purge to get rid of extra calories)...

3. Binge Eating disorders (People with *binge-eating disorder* often consume unusually large amounts of food and are unable to stop eating).

All these can occur when we are unable to fulfill our basic needs of body nourishment.

When our Root Chakra is healthy and balanced, we feel secure and have a strong desire to eat and live. When Root Chakra is strong then

1. We can focus on our set goals.
2. We develop an excitement for life.
3. We develop the courage to face any challenges of life.
4. We have a sense of security and a feeling of belonging to this world.

This is the foundation for building self-esteem and self-worth.

Ways of Healing Root Chakra

Gemstone Healing

Gems like Garnet, red jasper, black tourmaline, and bloodstone can be used to heal this chakra. These can be either worn in the form of rings or lockets or can even be placed on the root chakra area.

Exercises

People who have pain in the lower back or pelvic region should take up exercises for healing both.

Diets

Diets rich in red foods should be included like strawberries, tomatoes, beets, and pomegranate to heal this chakra.

Walking

Walking barefoot with awareness on the floor so that we can notice how our foot touches the ground and leaves the ground. We can also do hiking, gardening, swimming, etc.

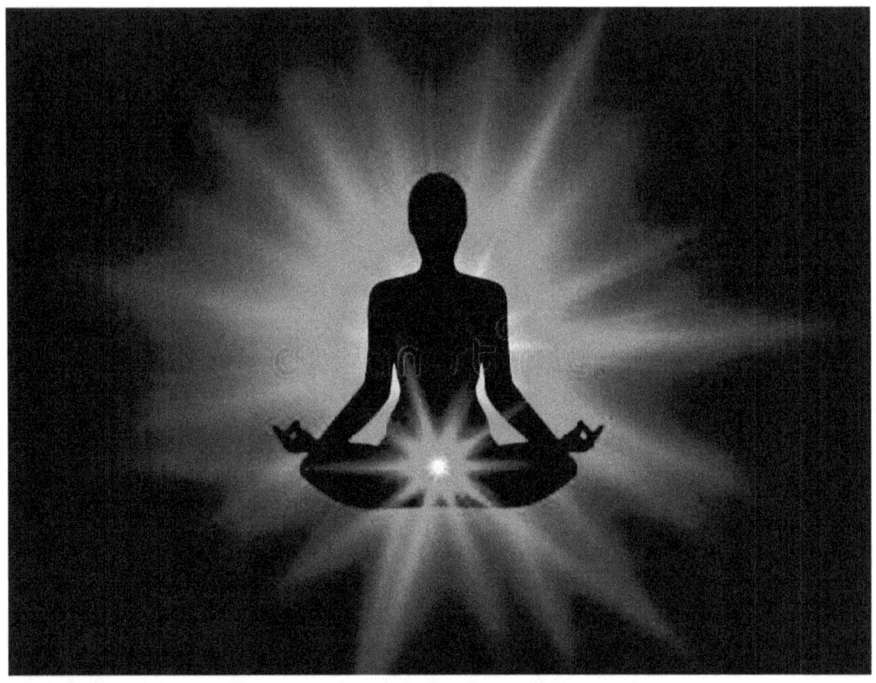

Muladhara

Besides this, we can do

1. Meditation

2. Reiki healing

3. Sound vibrations which are associated with this chakra.

YOGASANA FOR HEALING THIS CHAKRA

SUKHASANA

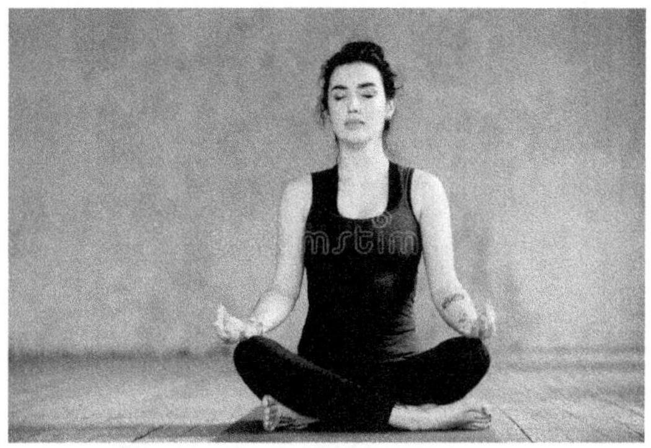

Sukhasana Fig 1

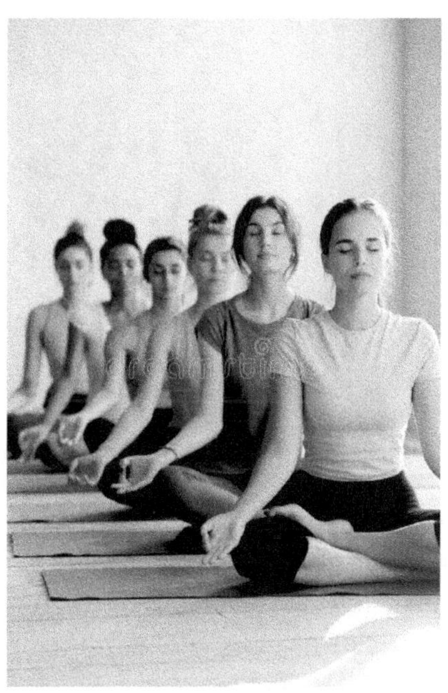

Sukhasana Fig 2

Seat yourself by squatting and closing your eyes. Feel the earth beneath you. Feel every part of your body touching the ground and experience the exchange of energy between the earth and you. Take a deep breath and exhale and feel every part of your body releasing to the ground. You experience the inner spine becoming lighter and the lift from the root of the tailbone to the crown of the head.

BALASANA

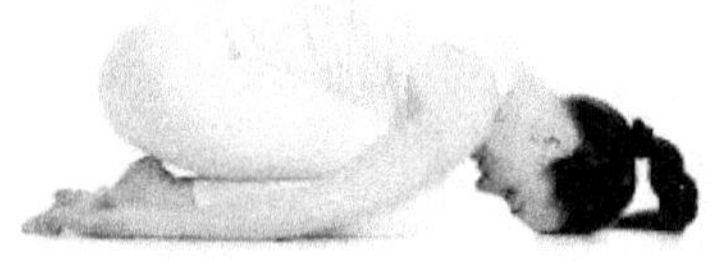

Balasana Fig 1

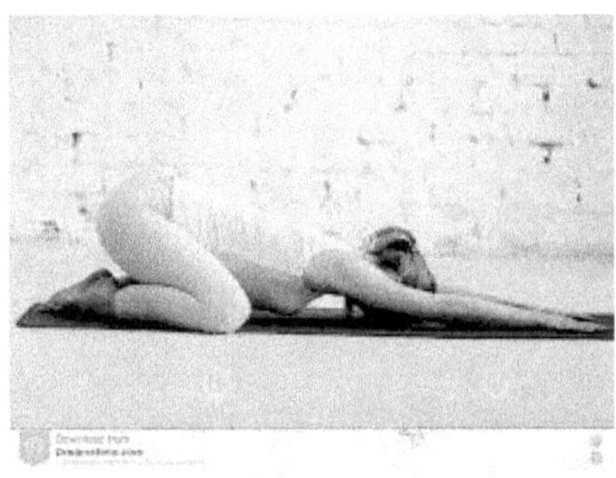

Balasana Fig 2

Sit in Dandasana and forward your hands and knees and then ease the sit bones back into the heels into a child pose. Then release your forehead to the ground and take 5 slow breaths. Allow your body to relax deeply and feel complete surrender and support.

TRIKONASANA

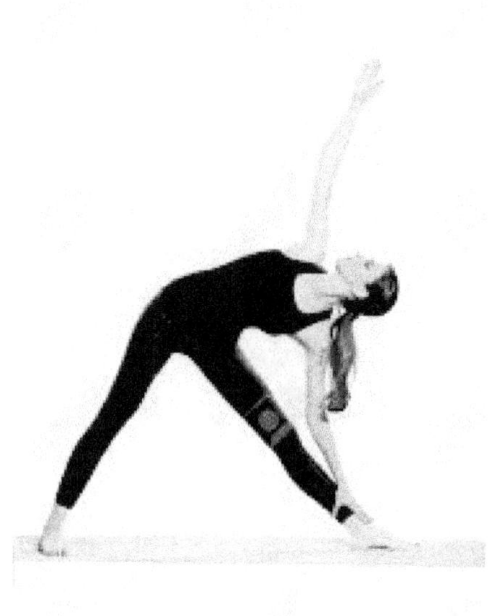

Trikonasana Fig 1

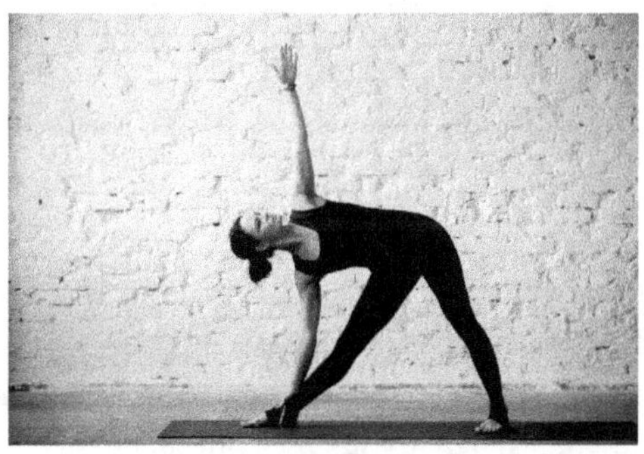

Trikonasana Fig 2

Spread your legs apart and your arms then bend down towards your right lengthening your right arm and torso over the right leg. Firm your feet down to the floor and extend your left arm upwards from the core of your heart. Repeat this for the other side also.

Commit yourself to root down through your feet and leg and feel the spaciousness these roots bring to the inner body.

MALASANA

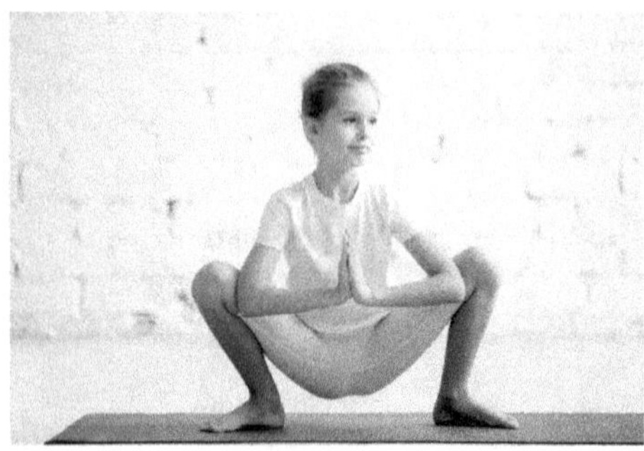

Malasana Fig 1

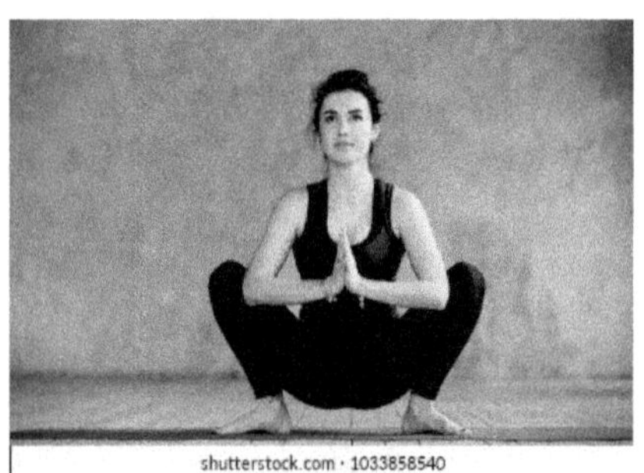

Malasana Fig 2

Squat deeply and feel yourself close to the ground.

Stand with feet slightly wider than hips and bend your knees lowering sit bones towards your heels. Turn your feet out as needed so that your knees and feet point in the same direction. You can even touch your hands to the ground till you feel stable.

Lengthen your spine and sit in an upright posture. Bring your hands together in Anjali mudra.

Widen the collar bones and press elbows towards the inner knees and bring your tailbone down.

Ardha Hanumanasana (Hamstring Stretch)

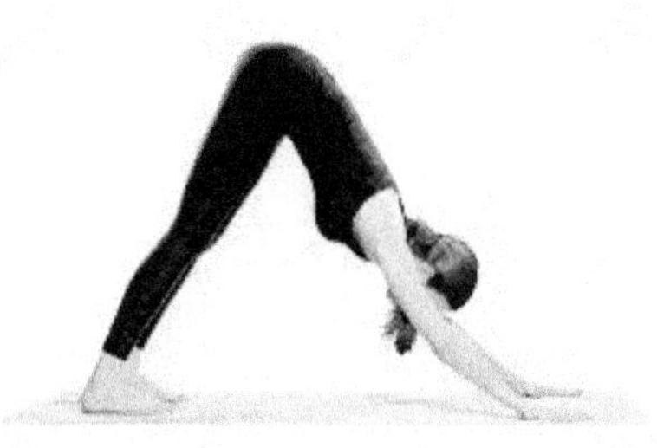

ADHO MUKHASANA

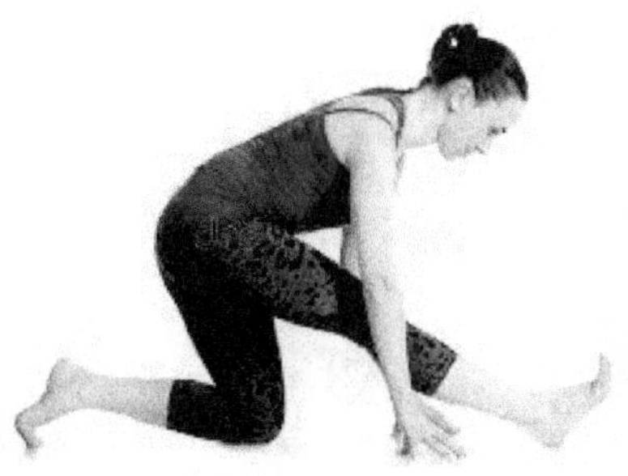

Hanumanasana

From Adho Mukhasana, move the right foot forward between both the hands and place the left knee gently on the ground, and pull the hips back.

Keeping your hips square and hands on the ground extend your spine. Move your inner spine forward and up and feel the legs and hips touching the earth and then draw back. Take 5 deep breaths and then change sides.

Besides these, other yoga asanas that help to align and open the Muladhara are

1. **Pavanamuktasna** – knee to chest pose.

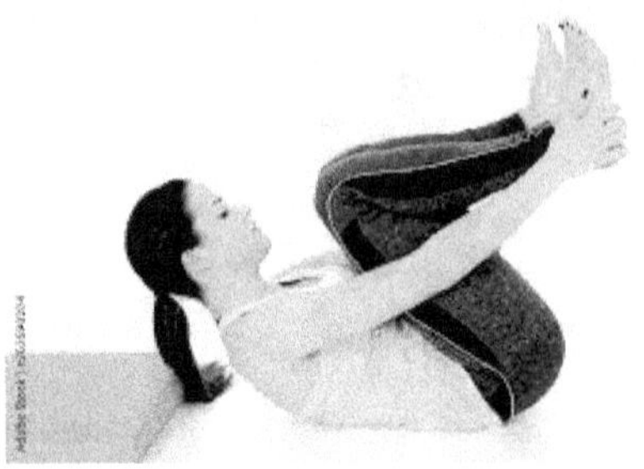

Pavanamuktasana

1. **Padmasana** – Lotus flexion.

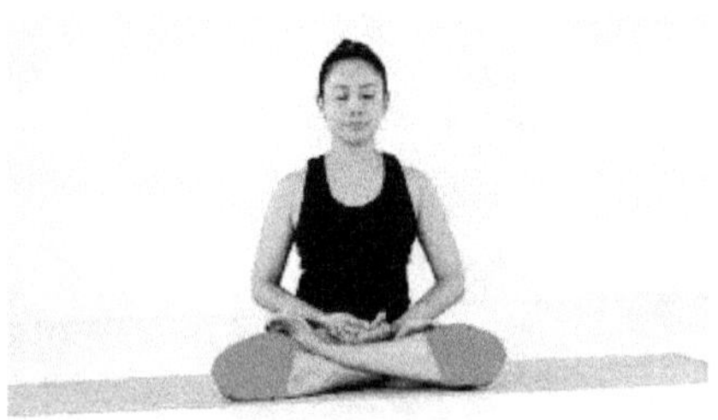

Padmasana

3. **Janu Sirsasana** – Head to Knee Pose

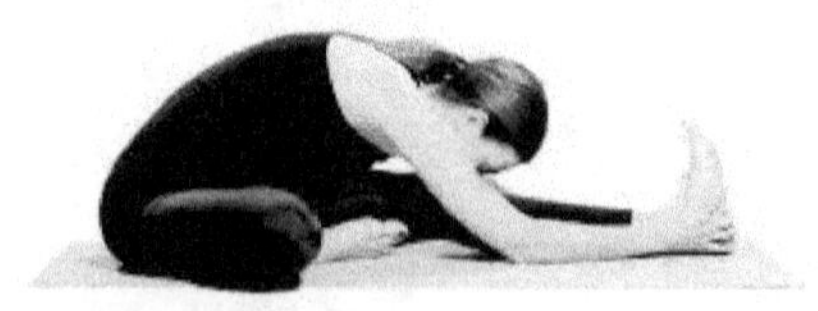

Janu Sirsasana

Bandha Yoga can be done by both Men and Women where you lock and tighten certain areas of your body which brings strong energy and strength to the first chakra.

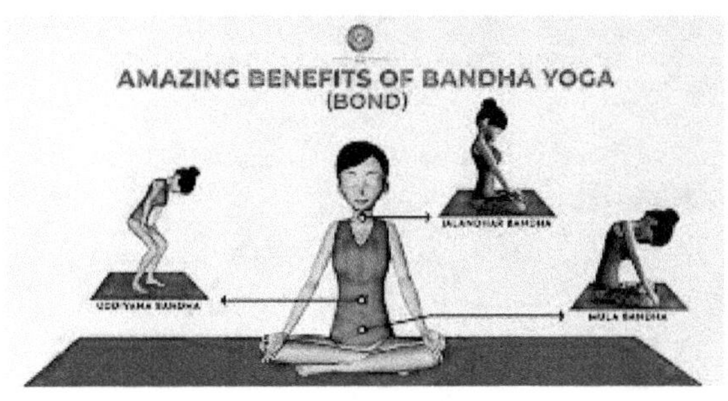

Bandha Yoga

Note: Chanting or toning sounds can also balance this chakra. The vibrations of this sound help the cells work in synchronization. This mantra is LAM.

For this, you have to sit silently and chant the mantra LAM visualizing the red color at the base of tail bone becoming bigger and bigger and radiating its energy to the entire body.

SUMMARY

1. Root Chakra is at the base of spine and is red in color. It is associated with the Earth.
2. With Root chakra you get strength to face challenges in life.
3. If Root Chakra is misbalanced, we are distracted and do not feel connected to the world.
4. Root Chakra when misbalanced leads to depression, constipation, loss of self-esteem, suicidal thoughts, eating disorders etc.
5. To balance Root chakra, we can use stones like Red jasper, Garnet and blood stone.
6. We can do meditation and chant mantra LAM

We can do Yogasanas like Malasana, Sukhasana, Ardha Hanumanasana, Trikonasana etc.

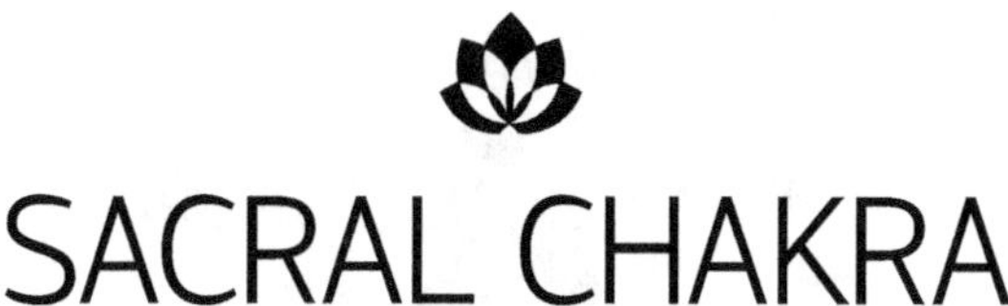

CHAPTER THREE

SACRAL CHAKRA

This Chakra is also called Swadishthana Chakra. It is located two inches below the belly button. It is orange in color and is associated with water.

This Chakra is associated with the Endocrine glands, Ovaries, and Testis. This Chakra is motivated by Pleasure and Joy. It is responsible for the enjoyment of life through the senses and also creates the foundation for emotional well-being.

Location	Below Belly Button
Color	Orange
Element	Water
Emotion	Pleasure and Joy and emotional well being
Seed Mantra	VAM

Swadishthan Details

hen it comes to sensuality, it helps us understand and develop intimate connections with others.

When it comes to creativity, it awakens creative expression, allowing to explore new ideas and stimulate the imagination.

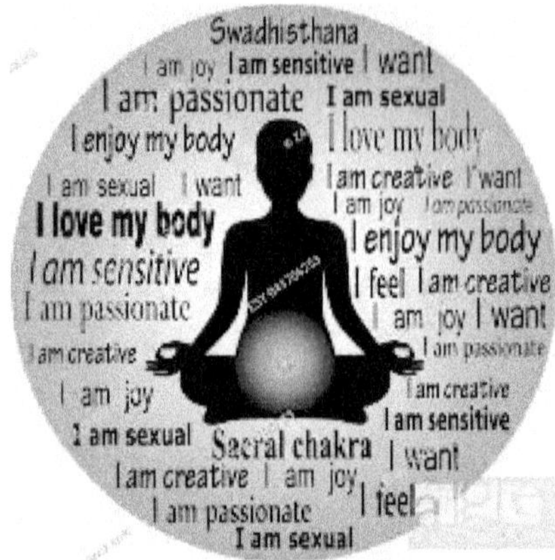

Sacral chakra

Due to the energy of this chakra, we can discover and explore our passion and this helps us enjoy life fully.

This chakra helps us feel connectivity, sexuality, maintains the quality of Interpersonal relationships, and also gives pleasure and contentment in life.

When this Chakra is blocked, then one suffers from fear that cannot be managed.

Mostly our Chakras are blocked due to factors like diet, negative thoughts, stress, attitude, physical impact, or a sedentary lifestyle.

Our Energies are imbalanced by repressing our emotions, lack of present-mindedness, resisting certain experiences.

Energy has a nature to flow and if it is blocked, it creates physical, emotional, and psychological sickness.

The Symptoms of a Weak Sacral Chakra are:-

1. Not allowing you to be emotionally and sexually intimate.

2. Eating disorders, addictions, low self-esteem, and dependency.

3. Low libido (sexual desire) and unbalanced emotions.

4. Feeling of confusion, abuse and hurt.

5. Kidney problems, UTI (Urinary Tract Infection), Chronic lower back pain.

6. Infertility, Sexual disorder, and gynecological problem.

7. Distrust for being loved.

8. A struggle for a healthy self-image.

9. Problems with the Intestine, gall bladder, and spleen.

10. Unsuccessful relationships.

Signs of imbalance:

Addictive behaviors, dysfunction, of sexual organs, fear of any change, instability of emotions.

In the body, the sacral chakra connects with reproductive issues (infertility, impotence, or menstrual issues) and lower back kidney, or stomach disorders.

Healing Methods

1. Healing with Mudras (using hand and finger gestures).
2. Do Meditation and Visualizations.
3. Use Mantra Chanting.
4. Yoga Postures.
5. Affirmations
6. Chakra Stones and Crystals
7. Color Therapy
8. Chakra Massage
9. Aroma Therapy
10. Sound and Music.

The Changes in thoughts and behavior can also speed up the process of healing the Chakra and give long-term benefits.

Burn Swadishthana incense and essential oils

Aromatherapy has a strong healing power to help restore feelings of sensuality and creativity. To open the sacral chakra, try to burn cleansing aromas like cardamom, eucalyptus, chamomile, spearmint, patchouli, ylang-ylang, rose, or clary sage.

Yoga for Sacral Chakra

1. Baddha Konasana (Butterfly Pose)
2. Upavishta Konasana (Wide-Angle Seated Forward Bend)
3. Pelvic Lifts
4. Kundalini Lotus
5. Sufi Grind (Seated Pelvic Circles)
6. Goddess Pose (Utkata Konasana)
7. Reverse Warrior Pose (Viparita Virabhadrasana)
8. Seated Forward Bend (Paschimottanasana)

Baddha Konasana

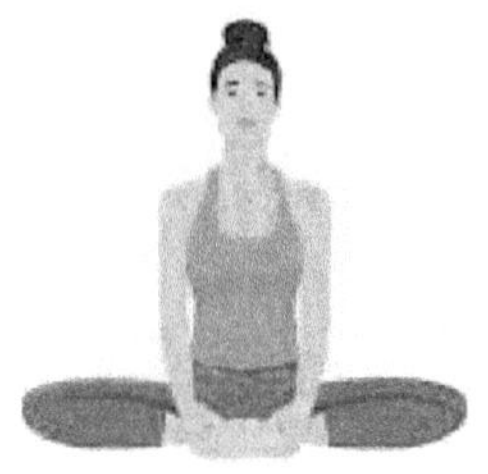

Baddha Fig1

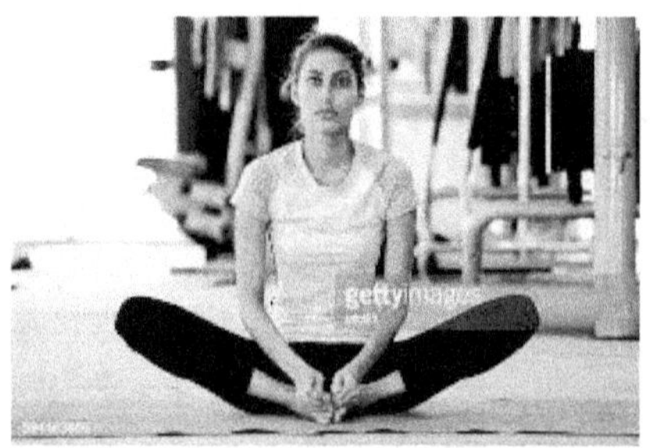

Baddha Fig2

1. Bring the soles of both the feet together in the seated position, such that they are close to the pelvis and allow the knees to fall on sides.

2. Ground the sit bones with the spine erect.

3. Press the soles together while holding your toes.

4. Try folding forward from the hip, keeping your spine long and erect and collar bones spread.

5. Stay in this position for 5 to 10 breathes.

6. Then sit straight lift your knees and straighten the legs.

Benefits

1. Increases hip mobility and stretches inner thighs.

2. Grounding and Calming.

Upavishta Konasana

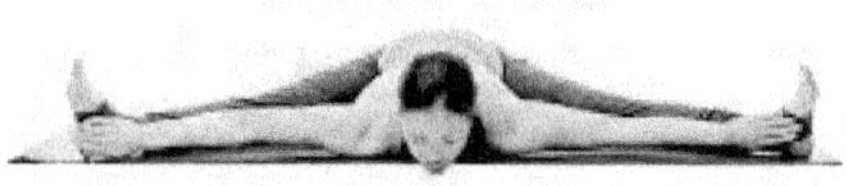

Upavishta Fig 1

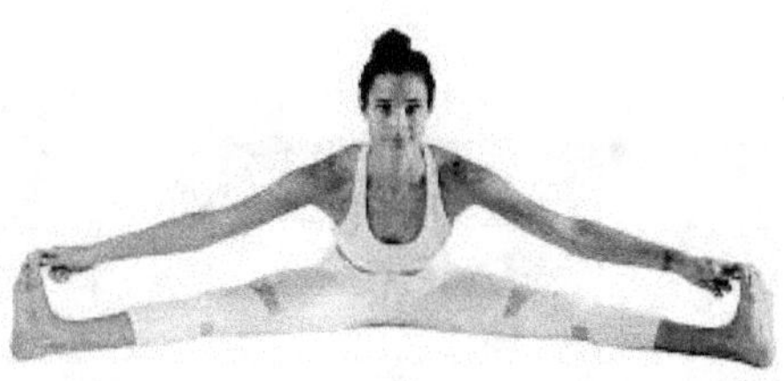

Upavishta Fig 2

1. Sit in Dandasana, and then spread your legs apart, till you feel, stretch and maintain a straight spine without falling back.

2. Flex your feet and keep your knees and toes pointing upwards facing the ceiling. Press your legs and sit bones and lengthen your spine.

3. With a straight spine, bend from the hips and place your hands between your legs on the floor and slowly exhale out as you put your hands forward.

4. Maintaining length, try not to arch, keep your spine erect in this bending position.

5. When you come out of this position, press your sit bones down as you exhale.

Benefits

1. It opens the hips and back of the body.

2. Stretches hamstrings and inner thighs.

3. Strengthens spine.

4. stimulates abdominal organs.

PELVIC TILT

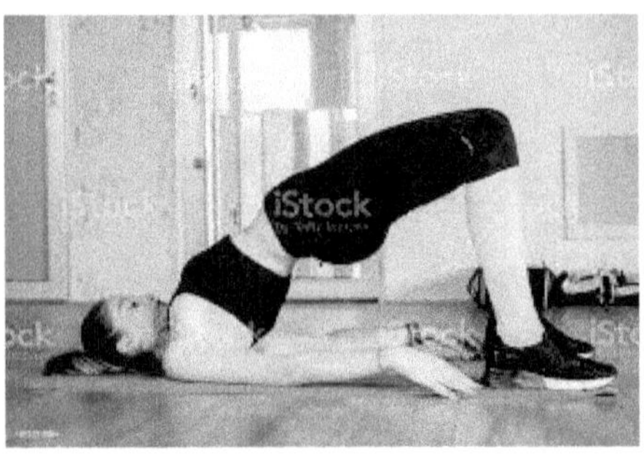

Pelvic tilt Fig 1

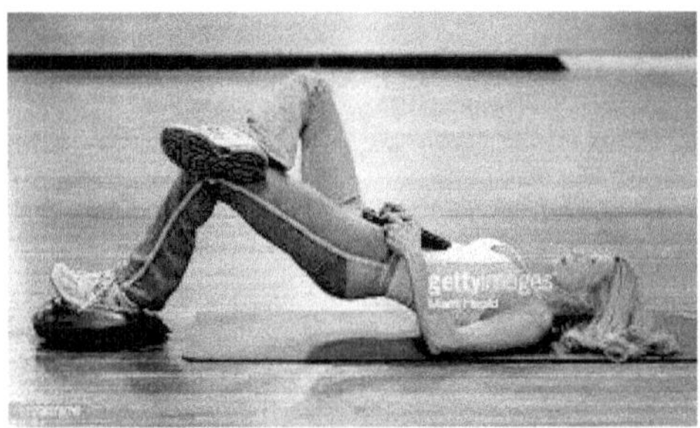

Pelvic tilt Fig 2

Through this yoga, the abdominal muscles are strengthened. First, we need to lie on our back on the floor and bend our knees. It is necessary to keep our back flat against the floor and tighten the abdominal muscles. Now we need to bend our pelvis slightly up. Hold for 10 seconds and repeat.

Benefits

This exercise helps to give strength to abdominal muscles and stretches the muscles in your lower back.

Kundalini Lotus Pose

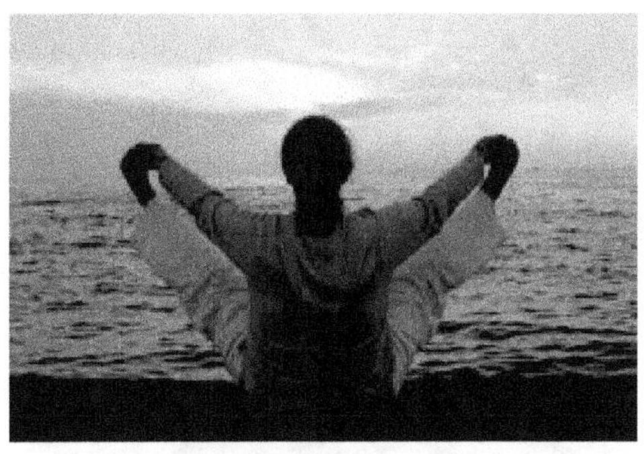

Kundalini Fig 1

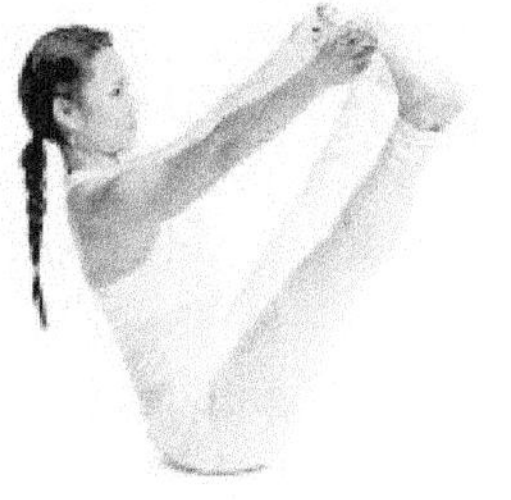

Kundalini Fig 2

In this yoga, we have to balance the sacrum and grasp the big toes. Then, holding the big toes, we need to raise the legs to 60 degrees from the floor and spread them wide apart such that the knees are not bent.

Benefits

This pose increases circulation in the lumbar spine and helps nourish and tone the abdominal organs. It also strengthens the ankles and legs and increases flexibility in the hips.

SUFI GRINDS

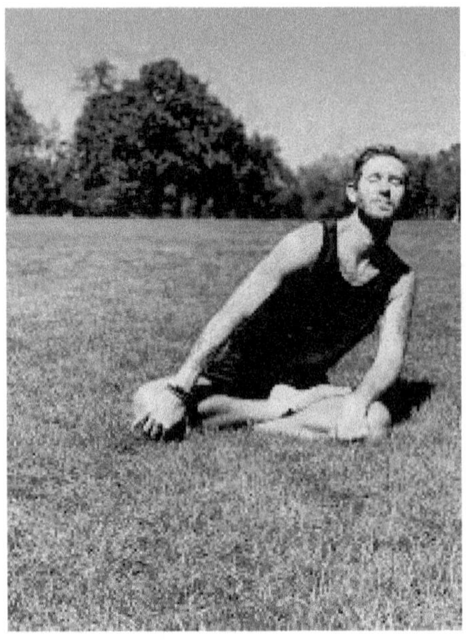

Sufi grinds Fig1

It is also known as seated torso circles or Kundalini circles. It is a seated yoga exercise for Therapeutic benefits. It is inspired by a peaceful and mystical sect of Islam.

First, sit in Sukhasana, then move the torso in circles around the middle line, inhaling as the body moves forward and exhaling backward. Practice in a clockwise and anti-clockwise direction for 3 minutes on each side.

Benefits

It improves mobility in the hips and spine. It also energizes the body and mind. It brings focus and awareness into the body, cultivating a sense of stillness.

It is useful in activating and balancing the lower chakras of the body. So our digestion is improved and treats the conditions affecting reproductive organs like endometriosis. It also gives a positive influence to adrenal gland maintaining stress levels.

Goddess Pose (Utkata Konasana)

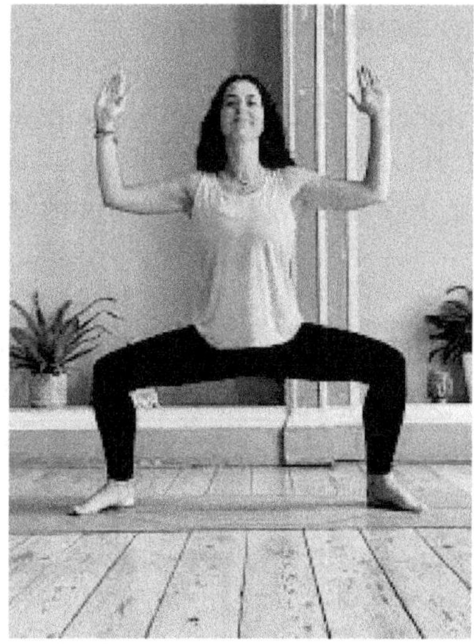

Utkata Fig 1

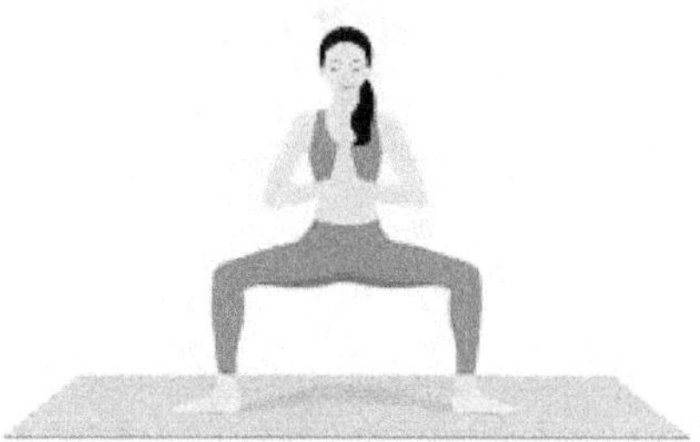

Utkata Fig 2

1. Stand straight and keep both the feet 3 feet apart. Bending the elbows at shoulder height, keep the palms facing each other. Turn both the feet out 45 degrees such that they face the corners of the room. While exhaling bend the knees over the toes squatting down.

2. Pressing the hips forward, keep the knees back. Now drop your shoulders down and back and press the chest to the front of the room. Keep your arms active, as if they were holding a big ball over your head. You need

to look straight ahead with the chin parallel to the floor.

Benefits and Contradictions of this Pose

Benefits: This pose helps to open the hips and chest. It also helps to strengthen and tone the lower body. It also stimulates the urogenital and respiratory systems. It is also useful for stimulating cardiovascular system.

Contraindications: Recent or chronic injury to the legs hips or shoulders.

Viparita Virabhadrasana

Benefits Reverse Warrior helps to strengthen the legs and open the side body. It also causes mobility in the spine, maintains balance, and also improves core strength. A good stretch is experienced in the front and rear thigh (quadriceps and hamstrings), hips, the muscles of the groin, and the intercostal muscles of the ribs.

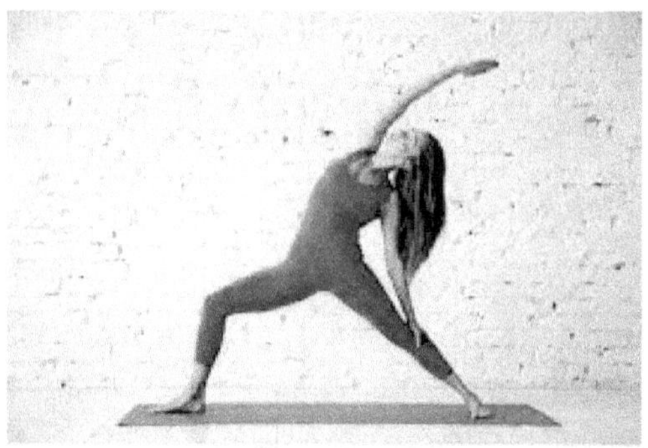

virbhadra Fig 1

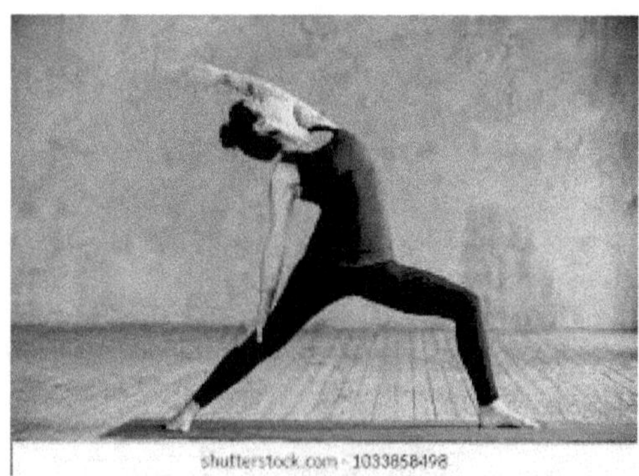

virbhadra Fig 2

When the sacral chakra is healthy, you will be able to experience and use energy for creativity, movement, procreation, desire, pleasure, and relationships. You can freely express your wants and needs in relationships, and pleasure will be a priority. You can easily tap into Creativity and visualization will become easy when the sacral chakra is balanced.

Paschimottanasana

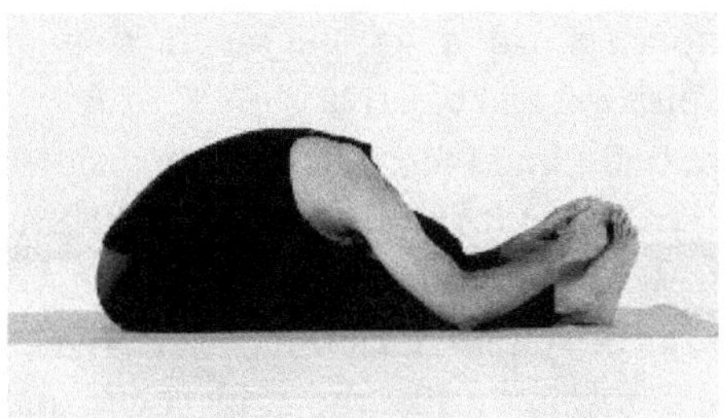

Paschimottanasana Fig 1

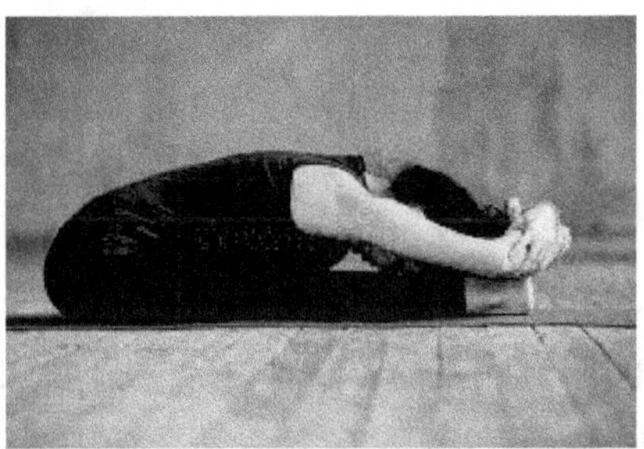

Paschimottanasana Fig 2

Spread your legs straight and stretch your arms forward to touch your feet, then bending your head move forward towards the foot, exhaling and remaining in this position for 5 breaths.

Reconnect with Water

Water is the chief element for sacral chakra and our ability to flow with change. We can spend more time with water by swimming, sitting near the sea or flowing stream, or we can also take a relaxing bath. There is a therapy known as Watsu, in which a person is gently held and guided in water. It is a powerful ritual for sacral healing.

Repeat positive affirmations about creativity.

By repeating affirmations, we intend to break old habits and adopt new ones. To open the sacral chakra, either repeat affirmations loudly, in your head or write them down. The affirmations are-

• I deserve to experience pleasure and all my needs are met.

• I attract relationships with loving, good people who will support me.

• I accept changes and make the best of my future.

• Every day, I experience more joy and satisfaction.

• I flow with inspiration and creativity.

• I have a vibrant body, and I feel comfortable inside it.

SOME OTHER WAYS TO BALANCE THE CHAKRA

1. **Off the Mat** – Wear Orange clothes while meditating and relaxing.

2. **Singing Mantras or sound vibrations** – The Vedic beej Mantra of this chakra is VAM. We can chant it like the Mantra OM and it works more on the same vibration frequency.

shakti1.jpg   3. **SHAKTI MUDRA**- keep your hands in front of

your chest, press the tips of the little finger and ring finger of both hands against each other Tuck your thumbs inside your palms, passing it through folded forefinger and middle finger. Then press the knuckles of both the middle and index finger of both hands and keep them separate.

4. Do Meditation

5. During the day drink a lot of water.

6. Move and dance more with hips and find some form of creative expression.

SUMMARY

1. Sacral Chakra is located two inches below the navel and is the center of creativity and sensuality.

2. It is orange in color and is associated with water.
3. When it is misbalanced then we develop eating disorders, distrust, kidney problems, infertility, etc.
4. To activate the chakra, we can do meditation and several Yoga postures like Baddha Konasana, Lotus Pose, Paschimottanasana, etc.
5. Do some affirmations and also resort to water therapies.

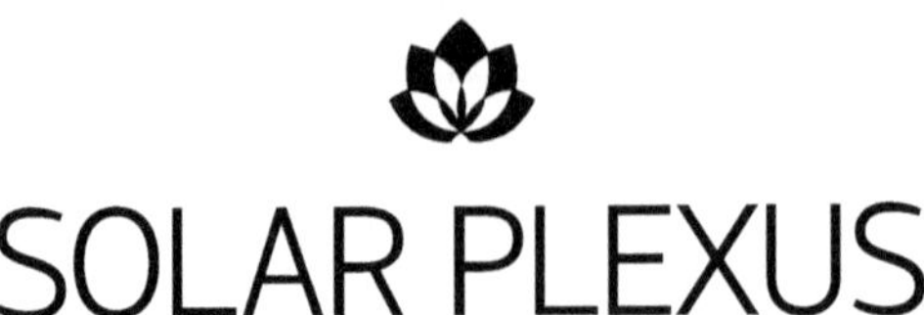

CHAPTER FOUR

SOLAR PLEXUS

It is also known as Manipura Chakra. It is present in the stomach area two inches above the navel. If this Chakra is active and balanced, we feel self-confident and develop a feeling of self-esteem as well as feel in control of life. The color of this chakra is Yellow.

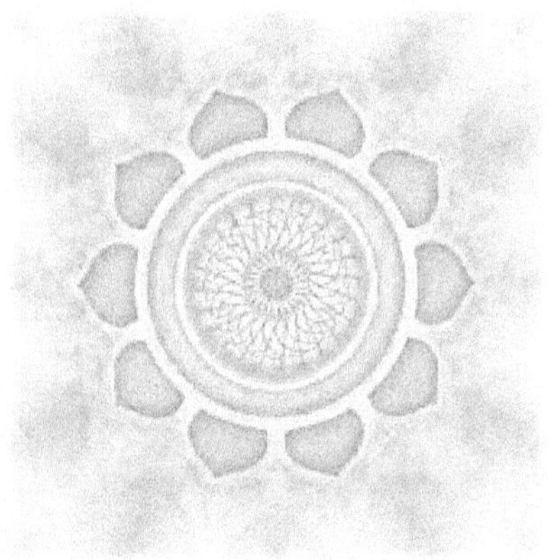

Solar Plexus

The word Manipura is taken from the Sanskrit word "Manipur" where Mani is a Jewel and Pur is a city so it is "City of Jewels". The Color of this Chakra is Yellow and the element associated with it is fire.

Being the house of fire or Agni and vital wind, it handles digestion and metabolism. The inward and outward flowing energy i.e. Prana and Apana Vayu meet together at a point in a balanced system.

Location	Two inches above the navel
Color	Yellow
Element	Fire or Agni
Emotion	Self-confidence and Self-esteem
Seed Mantra	RAM

Solar Plexus Detail

Manipura is the house of the celiac plexus (a large plexus of sympathetic nerves in the abdomen behind the stomach) which is responsible for most of the digestive system. It is related to Pancreas, Kidney, and adrenal functions.

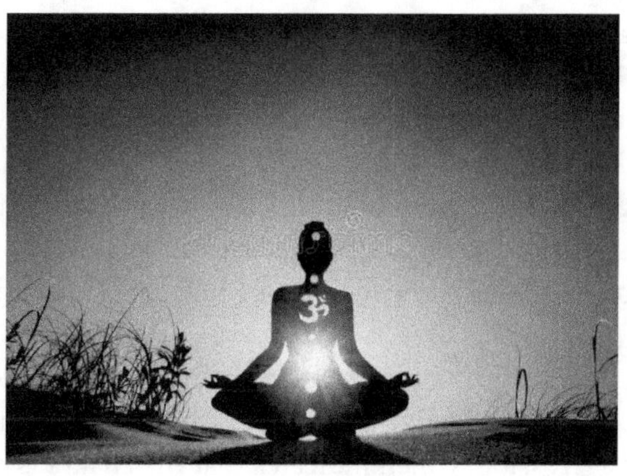

Solar Plexus Fig 2

Weak fire or Agni can lead to indigestion, misbalanced thoughts, and emotions which in turn can lead to toxicity i.e. ama.

Solar Plexus is behind the navel and is associated with Sun (Surya) Chakra which absorbs and assimilates Prana from the Sun. Since it is associated with sight, it is related to the eyes. It is also associated with feet, so helps in movement.

In the endocrine system, Solar Plexus is associated with Pancreas and outer adrenal glands. These glands secrete digestive hormones responsible for converting food to energy for the body. In the same way, Manipura radiates Prana throughout the body.

The Seed Mantra is – RAM

Gland – Pancreas

Psychological functions – Anger, Ego, and depression.

When this Chakra is balanced, then a person feels motivated, confident, and has a purpose in life.

When surrounded with negative energy, he/she can suffer from low self-esteem, feel troubled while making decisions, and have control issues.

Imbalances caused in Solar Plexus can lead to fatigue, over-eating, overweight, especially around the stomach, digestive system problems, hypoglycemia, and diabetes.

Characteristics

Yellow color is the symbol of energy and also connects a person with the Sun and Fire. This color represents rebirth, new beginnings, and Youth. The color yellow helps us connect to intellect and knowledge. People, who like yellow color, are associated with intellectual pursuits.

Manipura, being associated with fire, represents the energy of the Sun. The element fire kindles consciousness that gives us the motivation to strive for wealth and good health.

• Spending too much time on this chakra can cause burnout. If this chakra is not developed, then a person is fearful, weak, and becomes inert.

• The heart chakra receives feelings of love and compassion from this chakra.

• The fire energy helps in digestion and also absorbs nutrients.

• If this chakra has excessive fire, then it can lead to impulsive reactions like anger and aggression, which indicates that the chakra is blocked.

SIGNS OF BLOCKED CHAKRA

1. Digestive Issue.

2. Constipation.

3. Irritable Bowel Syndrome.

4. Eating disorders, Ulcers.

5. Diabetes

6. Issues with Pancreas, Liver, and Colon

7. Severe Emotional Problems

8. Doubt and mistrust of People.

9. Worries.

10. Low self-esteem, searching for continuous approval from others, which leads to unhealthy attachments to people or in life.

11. Victim to mentality, neediness, and lack of direction and self-esteem to stand up and take action.

UNBLOCKING MANIPURA

When Manipura is unblocked, it removes insecurity, leading to recognition of inherent power. You connect with the purpose of life which helps to have a better understanding of one's contribution to gaining success. This brings prosperity to personal and professional life.

Let go of negative things and dependency on others is reduced. There is a marked improvement in recognizing self-worth rather than focusing on material things. Positive Transformation is possible through consistent practice to investigate and identify the symptoms of blockage.

Well-balanced Solar plexus helps us effectively plan and achieve success. Cleaning and Opening this Chakra can make a person a good leader and create an inspiring life.

AFFIRMATIONS

1. I feel calm, confident, and powerful.
2. I feel ready to face challenges.
3. I feel motivated to pursue my purpose.
4. I am ambitious and capable.
5. I forgive myself for past mistakes and learn from them.
6. The only thing I need to control is how to respond to situations.
7. I can create positive change in my life.
8. I stand in my power.

YOGA FOR BALANCING

As Solar Plexus is associated with fire or Sun, the Sun provides healing energy.

Exercising or walking for 20 to 30 minutes in the Sun every day will fill every space and cell. If you cannot go out, try to visualize the Sun, feel its warmth and light power.

Yoga Poses

Paschimottanasana

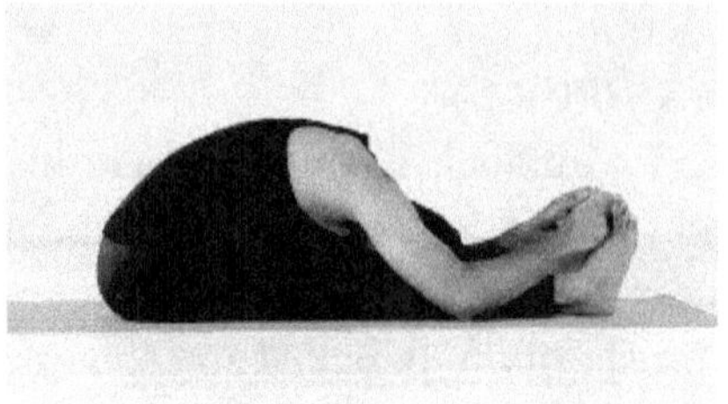

Paschimottanasana Fig 1

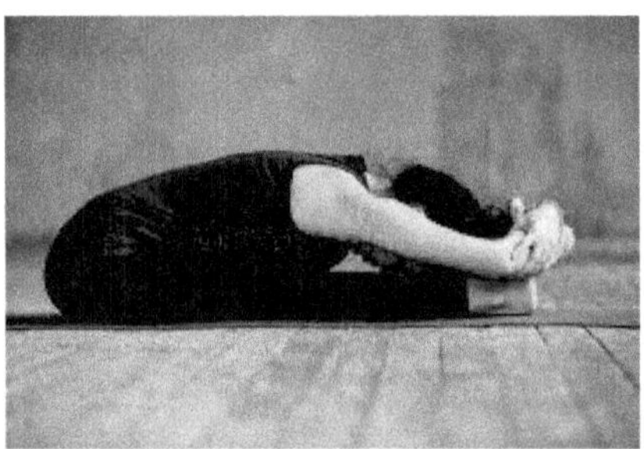

Paschimottanasana Fig 2

This is forward bending which is useful for digestion. This stimulation is caused by improved blood circulation and restores the best functional capacity of the spleen, liver, pancreas. This asana increases digestion and prevents constipation. If Manipura is activated, nutrients are absorbed easily.

Dhanurasana

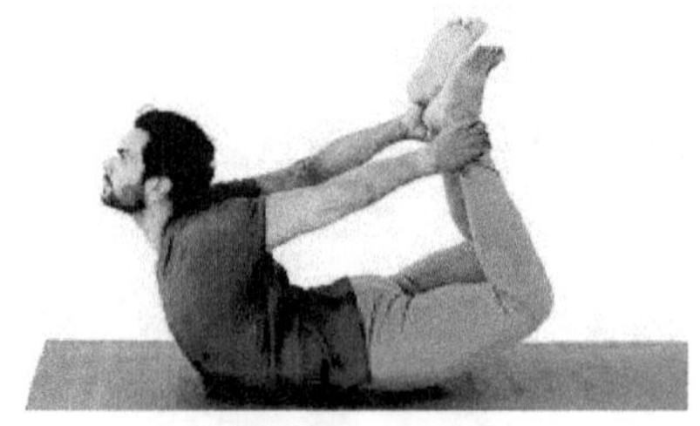

Dhanurasana Fig 1

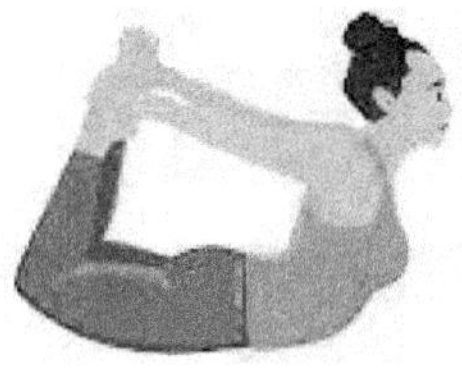

Dhanurasana Fig 2

This is a back-bending pose that gives enormous massage to various organs of the digestive system, particularly the liver and pancreas.

This helps in the elimination of toxins and waste and helps in better digestion. The extension of the neck stimulates the thyroid gland promoting healthy secretion of hormones, which improves metabolism for ideal body weight management.

Ardha Matsyendra/Half Spinal Twist

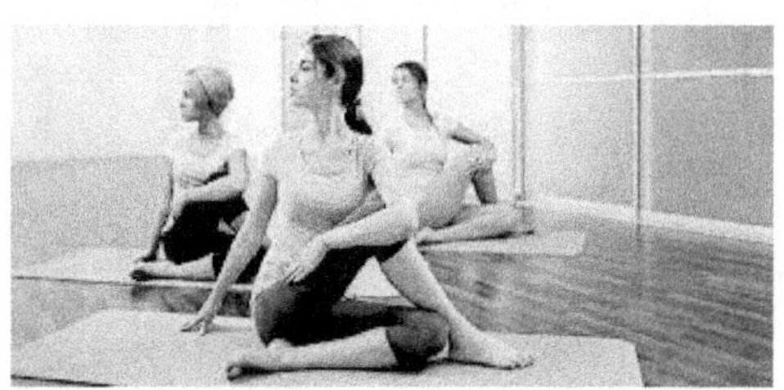

Spinal Twist Fig 1

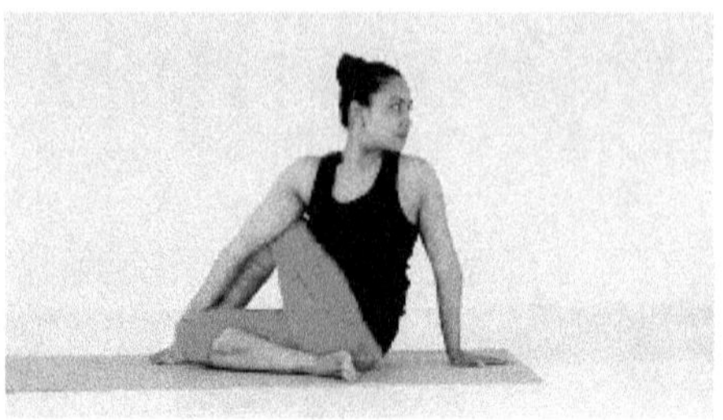

Spinal Twist Fig2

This stimulates the digestive system, liver, and gall bladder and helps in detoxification, and improves digestion.

Bhujangasana

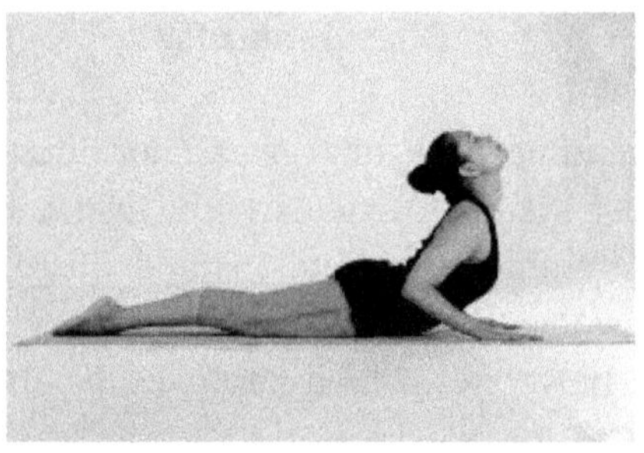

Bhujangasana Fig 1

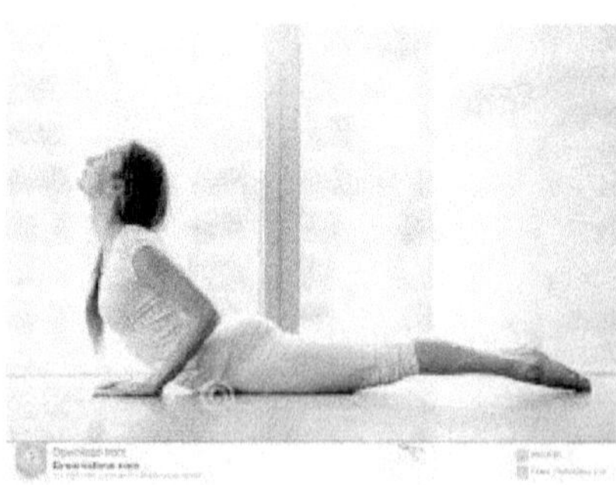

Bhujangasana Fig 2

1. First lie down on your stomach and keep your toes flat on the floor, make sure that your soles face upwards, and rest your forehead on the ground.

2. Try keeping your legs together with your heels and feet touching each other.

3. Keep both palms on the ground beneath your shoulders.

4. Take a deep breath, and slowly lift your head, chest, and abdomen keeping your navel on the floor.

5. Putting equal pressure on both the Palms, pull your torso back and off the floor, using both hands.

6. Arch back as much as possible and tilt your head back and look up.

7. Maintain this pose while breathing evenly for 4 to 5 breaths.

8. Now breathe out and bring your abdomen, chest and head back to the floor and relax.

9. Repeat 4-5 times.

Benefits

1. It opens up the shoulder and neck to relieve pain.

2. Tones abdomen.

3. Strengthens the entire back and shoulders.

4. Improves flexibility of the upper and middle back.

5. Expands chest.

6. Improves blood circulation.

7. Reduces fatigue and stress.

8. Useful for people with respiratory disorders like asthma.

The Seed Mantra

The seed Mantra is RAM. This reminds the Yogi that they can connect to their power without force by letting go.

SUMMARY

1. This Chakra is located two inches above the navel and is responsible for digestion and metabolism.

2. The Color Associated with it is Yellow and the element associated is fire.

3. Cleaning and opening this chakra can make a person a good leader and create an Inspiring life.

4. For its best functioning, walk for 20-30 minutes in the sun.

5. The Mantra related to it is RAM.

6. Yogasanas are Bhujangasana, Ardhamatsyasana, and Paschimottanasana etc.

7. If this Chakra is blocked it can lead to Constipation, Diabetes, Severe Emotional Problems, Worries, mistrust, and doubt in People.

CHAPTER FIVE

HEART CHAKRA

It is also known as **Anahata Chakra.** It is located at the center of the spine at heart level. Anahata means 'unhurt'. It acts as an individual's center of empathy, compassion, love, and forgiveness.

Name in Sanskrit – Anahata means unstruck sound also translated as "pure" or "unhurt".

Location	Heart
Element	Air
Color	Green
Emotions	Love, Fear, hate
Seed Mantra	YAM

Heart chakra details

From Manipura, the energy flows upwards and manifests in 3 forms- fear, love, and hatred. The sensation is felt in the heart region.

When you feel the following

1. Scared, fearful, hateful, panicked, horrified and hostile.
2. Loving, loved, tender, warm, devoted, adored or adoring.
3. Or Both.

These are all related to the heart chakra.

SIGNS OF BLOCKED HEART CHAKRA

Due to a blocked Heart Chakra, one can feel heartbroken, fearful, and unloved. This can have a big impact on the fourth chakra. When a person experiences love then there is no fear and if there is fear, one never experiences love.

People who fear sometimes have love. When love is prominent, there is no fear or hatred. When hatred becomes prominent, fear and love take a back seat, which means that people who are full of hatred, have no love or fear at all.

When this Chakra is aligned and in good condition, then you feel good and open, loved and loving and unconditional love flows through you.

Healing

To live a life full of unconditional love, it is necessary to heal the heart and get the energy flowing. This is a necessary ongoing practice. The chakras always want the energy to flow, move and be free.

Yoga Postures, Pranayamas, breathing techniques, and meditation will help energy flow upwards and thus balance your Chakras.

Some Yoga Postures are

1. Puppy Dog Pose (Anahatasana)
2. Camel Pose (Ushtrasana)
3. Wheel Pose (Chakrasana)
4. Upward-Facing Dog Pose (Urdhva Mukhasana)

Extended Puppy Pose

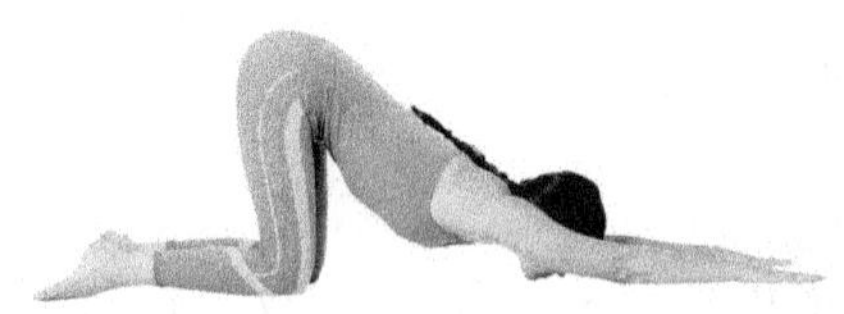

Puppy Pose Fig 1

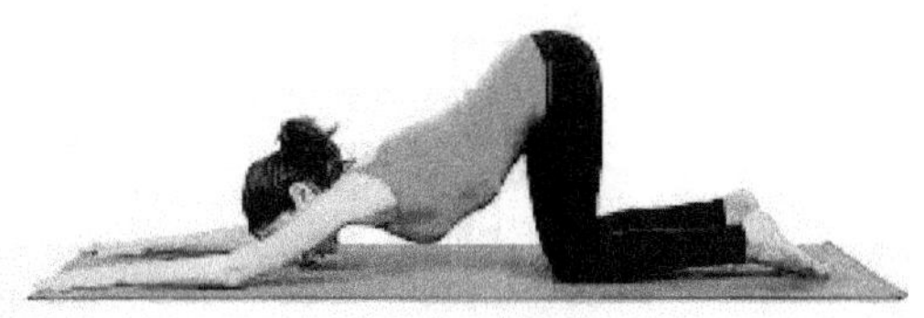

Enter Caption

Step 1

Come on all fours. Keep your shoulders such that they are above your wrists, hips, and your knees. Walk forward with your hands a few inches and curl your toes under.

Step 2

While exhaling, move your buttocks halfway backward and towards your heels. Your arms should be active, and don't let elbows touch the ground.

Step 3

Drop your head on the floor or blanket and let your neck relax. Keep a slight curve on the lower back. Press your hands to feel a nice stretch in your spine and stretch through your arms while pulling hips back towards the heels.

Step 4

Breathe into your back, feel the spine lengthen in both directions. Hold for 30 seconds to 1 minute and then release your buttocks down to your heels.

Camel Pose (Ushtra Asana)

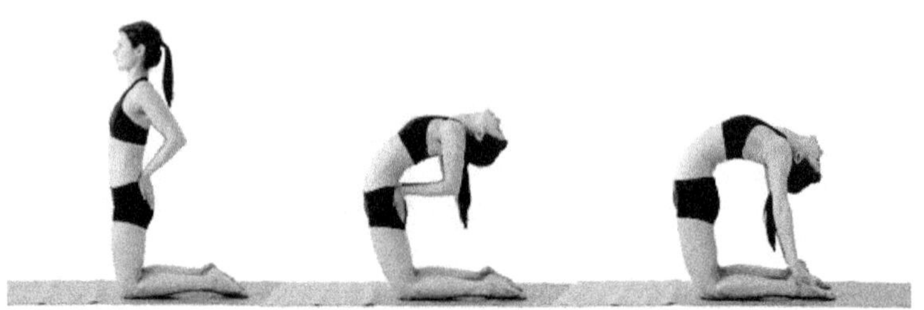

Camel Pose Fig 1

1. Kneel on the floor, keeping your hip wide apart in line with your shoulders. If you feel any problem with your knees, place a folded blanket on the Yoga mat underneath you. Keeps the thighs perpendicular to the floor with the soles of feet facing the ceiling.

1. Place your hands on the lower back such that the fingers face downwards.

3. While inhaling, draw in your tailbone towards your pubis to show as if your navel is pulling it. Arch your back reaching back to your heels, and straighten each arm to touch your soles.

4. Drop your head back. Remain in this state for 30 seconds.

5. To come out of this pose, exhale bringing down hour head towards your chest and your hands towards your hips. Engaging the lower belly, use your hands to support your lower back.

Benefits
1. Improves Digestion
2. Stretches and opens front of the body.
3. Tones abdominal organs.

4. Strengthens shoulder and back.

5. Relieves lower backache.

6. Improves posture and flexibility of the spine.

7. Alleviates menstrual discomfort.

Chakrasana

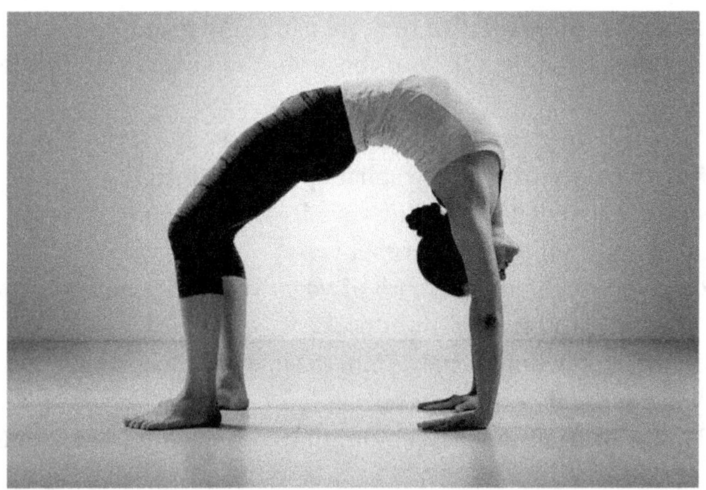

Chakra Fig 1

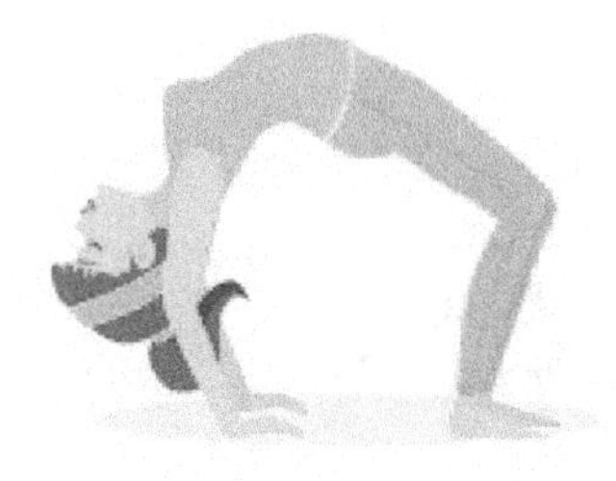

Chakra Fig 2

It is a back-bending posture that opens the chest, tones thighs, abdomen, and arms, and engages the whole body. It helps release sadness and depression.

Steps

1. Start by lying on your back.

2. Keep your feet flat on the floor and bend your knees. Keep your feet firm and at a distance such that they are parallel to the hips.

3. Place both hands on the floor above your shoulders with fingers facing down.

4. Now Press your hands and lift your upper body off the mat, such that the crown of your head should rest lightly on your mat.

5. Now Press your feet and lift your legs, pelvis, and abdomen off the mat, such that the inner thighs are active.

6. Push your feet, so that more of your weight is experienced in your palms. This will protect your lower back.

7. Continue pressing firmly into the mat to maintain strength and stability in your arms.

8. Hang your head in a neutral position, so that you do not strain your neck.

9. Hold for 5-10 breaths.

10. To come out of this posture, you can lower your arms and legs bringing your spine back onto the mat vertebrae by vertebrae.

Benefits of Chakrasana

• Increases energy and heat
• Strengthens the arms, legs, spine, and abdomen
• Opens the chest
• Stretches the shoulders
• Stretches the hip flexors and core
• Strengthens the gluts and thighs
• Increases flexibility in the spine

Upward Facing Dog Pose — *Urdhva Mukha Svanasana (OORD-vaa-MOO-kaa-shvaa-SUN aa)* —

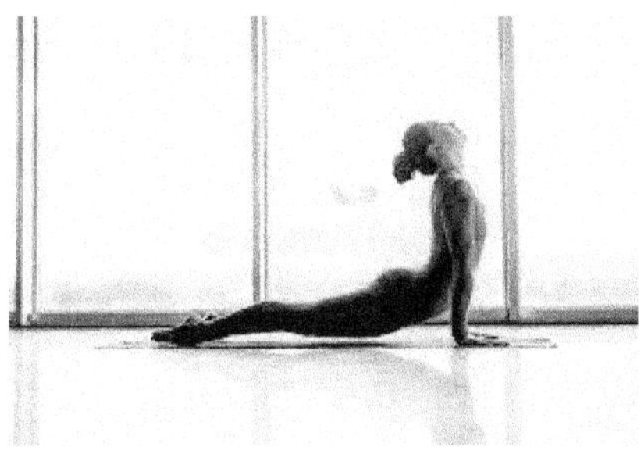

Urdhva Mukha Svanasana Fig 1

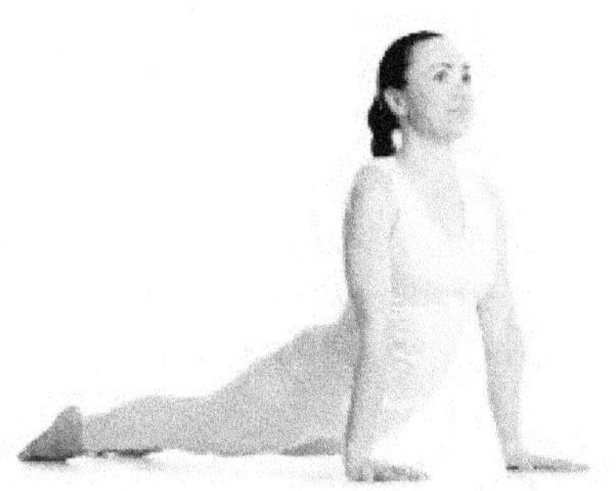

Urdhva Mukha Svanasana Fig 2

This back-bending posture gives strength to the arms, wrists, and spine. This pose helps to stretch back; as a result, the pain in the lower back is relieved. The Sanskrit words like Urdhva and mukha mean upward and face respectively. While svana and asana mean dog and pose respectively. So in all, it means upward-facing dog pose.

Step-by-Step Instructions

1. First, lie flat on your stomach keeping the soles of your feet such that they face upwards. Keep your arms straight beside your body.

2. Now bend your elbows and place your palms towards the side of the lower ribs.

3. Lift your upper body, hips, and knees off the mat while inhaling, putting pressure on your palms. This will make you feel that the entire weight of your body is on your palms and the top of your feet.

4. You can either look straight or slightly tilt your head upwards.

5. See that your neck is not strained and your writs are in line to the shoulders.

6. for 5-10 breaths, stay in this position

7. Gradually lower your knees, hips and torso on the mat when you exhale.

Benefits

• It helps to stretch and strengthen the back

• It gives relief in the lower backache.

• The arms and wrists are strengthened

• It helps to improve posture

The abdominal organs are stimulated.

Other Methods of Healing

For healing heart chakra, there are several holistic remedies that can help align the body, mind, and spirit. Some remedies are aromatherapy, sound healing, movement and color therapy, meditation, and crystal healing to re-establish harmony within the body-mind organism.

Meditation

Sit in a cross-legged comfortable position and close your eyes. When you feel completely relaxed, you can feel the green light from the heart chakra emerging and surrounding you. Allow this light to spread from the top of your head to your feet. Repeat this at least three times.

Crystal Therapy

The best method to heal any chakras is using a crystal as its vibrations have strong healing power. First, find a quiet place and then lie down by placing the crystal at the center of the chest. Let the vibrations of the crystal take away all the negative energies from the heart and fill it with positivity. After this remove the crystal and place it in a bowl of water to remove all negativity absorbed by the crystal and reenergize it.

Connect with nature:

Activities like gardening, biking, etc help us to remain close to nature. When you remain in close contact with nature, you feel the green light, emitting out and engulfing you.

If at times, your heart chakra is blocked, you need to be patient. Once your chakra is unblocked, you begin to love yourself more and new opportunities emerge in your life.

The seed mantra of the Heart chakra is **YAM**. This mantra helps us at

Spiritual and physical level. We feel more loved and improvement is felt in our relationships.

SUMMARY

1. Heart Chakra is also known as Anahata Chakra and is located towards the heart.
2. The color associated with it is green and the element is Air.
3. The emotions of love, fear and hatred originate from Solar Plexus and move towards the Heart Chakra.
4. To balance the heart chakra, we can do Yoga Poses like Chakrasana, Urdhvamukhasana, Ushtrasana, Anahatasana, etc.
5. We can do Crystal Healing and Meditation as well.
6. We can even spend time with Nature and experience green light emerging from the heart.
7. The Beej Mantra is YAM.

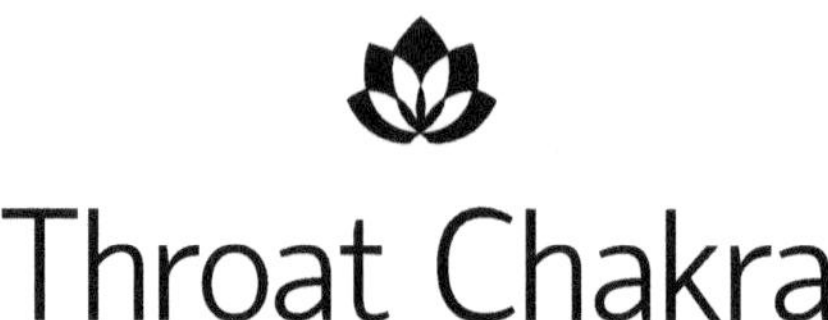

CHAPTER SIX

Throat Chakra

This is also known as Vishuddha Chakra. It is at the base of the throat. The color of this chakra is blue. The energy element associated with it is communication and the power to inspire and express.

Location	Base of throat
Color	Blue
Element	Communication
Seed Mantra	HAM

Throat chakra details

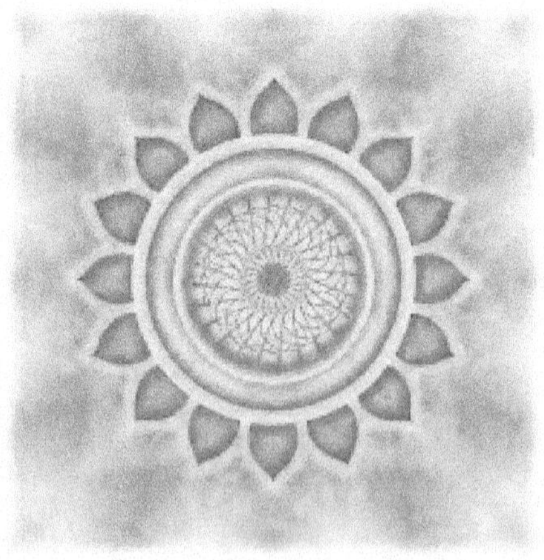

Throat chakra

This Chakra is blocked when we consume some unhealthy substances or come in contact with polluted air. When this chakra is active, we feel healthy. The word 'vishuddha' taken from Sanskrit actually means to detoxify mind and body and bring in purity.

Since the blue color is related to the Throat chakra, the energy of blue purifies, heals, and calms the mind and the person feels connected to the divine. When a person gets enough space and freedom, he can easily express his emotions.

Now, since we know that the blue color gives the power of communication, it further gives us the strength to speak the truth. Because of the energy of the blue color, the mind becomes still, and this is possible only when no negative thoughts clutter our mind. The seed mantra is HAM.

Let the Space expand your mind

This Chakra is associated with space and gives us the power to expand our thoughts and speak the truth. It helps us change our perception of life. We can understand others deeply. We get to know ourselves by feeling deeply connected to our inner selves. The divine power gives us guidance in every sphere of our lives.

Due to blocked throat chakra, the following can happen

- We might be afraid to speak out our personal truth.
- We might feel difficulty in expressing our thoughts.
- While speaking or communicating, we might become anxious.
- We might hesitate in expressing emotions
- We might find difficulty in searching for words to express your feelings
- People around us might misunderstand us.
- We might develop an aggressive behavior
- We might use negative words or do negative actions.

Since the vishuddha chakra is connected to the throat, we might experience physical problems when this chakra is blocked. We might feel sore throat, pain, or stiffness in the neck area. Our hormonal levels might fluctuate at times also.

In addition, according to Malaspina, we might either show sudden outbursts of emotions or might become extremely quiet.

Healing the Throat Chakra

Whenever we work on balancing the chakra, the chances of leading a happy and balanced life increase. It is easy to heal this chakra which might actually improve communication skills and this impacts all the aspects of our life. If this chakra is balanced, we get a feeling of freedom and the power to understand our own inner selves.

Yoga techniques to stimulate the Throat Chakra

The asanas of Yoga help to connect our spiritual and physical bodies. Concentrating on the breath while doing asana helps us release all tensions and this energizes the throat and thyroid. Following are the Yoga asanas to open the throat chakra.

- **.Shoulder stand | Sarvangasana-** This pose helps to stimulate the thyroid gland and activate the vishuddha chakra. Due to this asana, the blood flow and oxygen increase in the lungs. Due to better blood circulation, the digestive system also improves.

- **Plough Pose |Halasana** - This asana helps to calm the nervous system. It helps to reduce stress, fatigue, headaches. By doing this asana, the thyroid gland and abdominal organs are stimulated and thus help to remove blockage in the throat chakra.

Mindfulness Meditation

To connect with our inner truth, start by making your mind quiet. Focus your attention on the breath, which helps to calm thoughts. Inhale deeply and feel the flow of air passing through the lungs smoothly. When you exhale, feel the release of all negative energies and thoughts that clutter your mind.

Effective chakra foods

There are various foods to heal and balance various chakras of our body. Some specific dietary changes can be made to heal specific chakras. Fruits like apples, oranges, and all other fruits that grow on trees are associated with the healing of throat chakra. Some spices that can be added to food to heal the throat chakra are salt, ginger, and lemongrass.

Throat Chakra affirmations

There are certain affirmations that help to break old patterns and create effective new ones. There are some affirmations for throat chakra that help in effective and open communication. Some examples are

1. I feel comfortable speaking my mind.
2. I am a good listener.
3. I am confident while speaking.
4. I can express my thoughts clearly.
5. I can speak and listen in a balanced manner.

These affirmations will help us create new thought patterns and behaviors and even our actions are such that they help us in open self-expression.

Include the color blue in your life

According to certain Yoga teachers and reiki healers, since blue color is related to Throat Chakra, certain blue crystals like lapis lazuli, turquoise can help heal the throat chakra.

According to Guadalupe Terrones, since the throat chakra is related to sound, minerals effectively work with the throat chakra, since each mineral has a different resonating frequency.

If one wears a necklace of one of these gems, then it helps to heal the throat chakra.

2. Do neck stretches

To help balance the throat chakra, we can do neck stretches to open the area around the neck. Simple neck stretches help prevent help to cure stress and tension in the neck area.

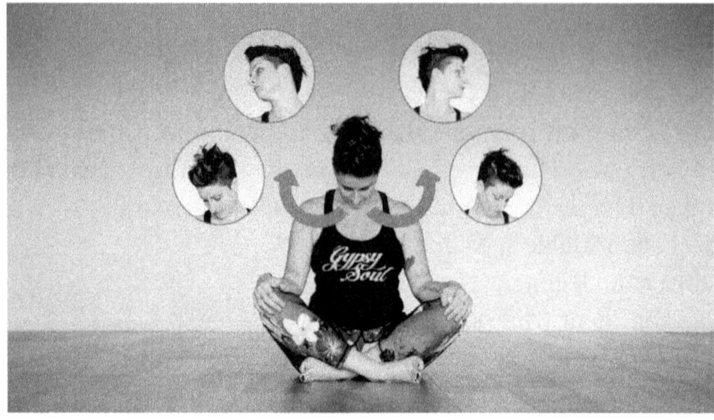

Neck stretch Figure

To do this stretch:

1. Drop your chin down toward your chest.

2. Tilt your head to the left. Relax your shoulders and the head should be tilted such that the left ear is close to your left shoulder. Doing this you can feel a stretch in the right side of your neck.

3. Remain in this position for 30 to 60 seconds. Then again move your head back down to your chest and then change to the opposite side and do the same.

Shoulder stand – Sarvangasana

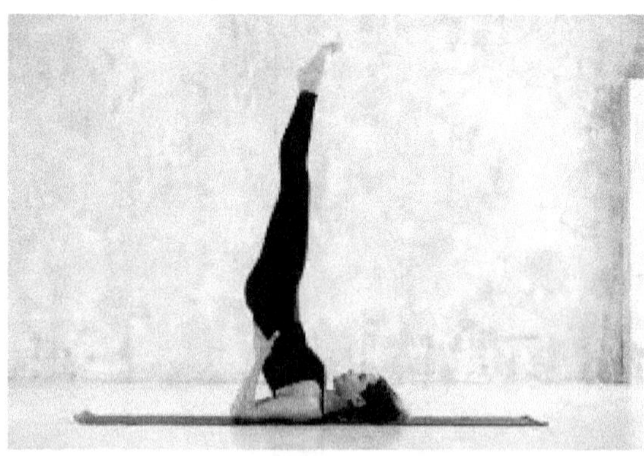

Sarvangasana Figure

The other name of this pose is Candle Pose and commonly known as 'Queen of asanas'. It is one of the most important Hatha Yogas and has various benefits on the entire body. The word Sarvang literally means 'all limbs'. So it has a positive effect on all parts of the body including thyroid gland. It also improves metabolism of the body.

Instructions to follow

1. Lie down with your back straight. Keep your feet together and your arms besides your body.
2. Breathe in and lift your legs to 90 degrees. Keep your neck and head on the floor.
3. Lift your hips up facing the ceiling and keep your hands on your hips.
4. Lift your hips higher and keep your chest towards your chin.
5. Maintain the pose by supporting your back with your hands. Make sure that your feet are above your head.
6. Breathe slowly in this position and focus on the throat region.

For coming out of this pose, slowly move your feet and drop them towards your head and remove your hands, keeping them on the floor, gently roll out of the pose.

Benefits of Shoulder stand

• It rejuvenates the Throat chakra and therefore helps in proper functioning of thyroid and Parathyroid glands. This helps improve metabolism, digestion and insulin production.

• It helps in reducing strain on your heart by slowing down the heart rate and blood pressure.

• The parasympathetic nervous system is activated, thus improving the digestive system and also helps in hormonal balance.

• It is useful for varicose veins and hemorrhoids as it improves blood circulation in the legs.

• This pose also helps in abdominal breathing rather than lung breathing.

• It helps in curing constipation and improves digestion.

• The heart and lung region get a gentle massage by this pose.

• It helps to give strength to the core muscles, the legs, buttocks, and lower back. It also helps in strengthening the upper back and arms.

Who should not try this Pose

People suffering from the following issues should avoid doing this Pose if they feel any discomfort.

• Hypertension

• Heart problems

• Neck or shoulder problems

• Those that had undergone recent surgery (eyes, ears, nose) or have inflammation in the head region.

• Those who have arthritis or osteoporosis

• Brain injuries

• Those that have pain in the lower back or have spinal problems

• Those that have migraine

• Asthma or other breathing disorders

HALASANA

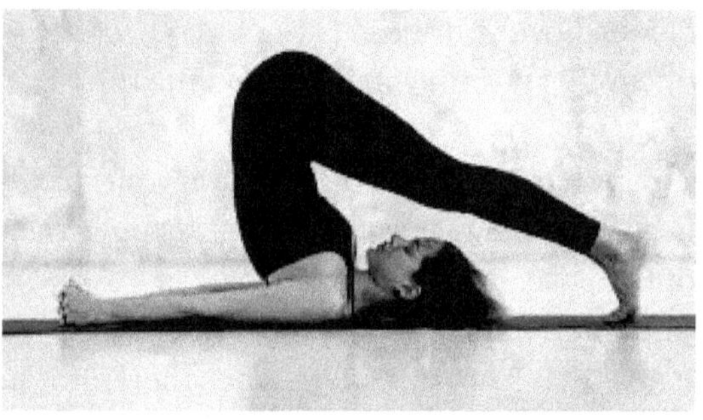

halasana Fig1

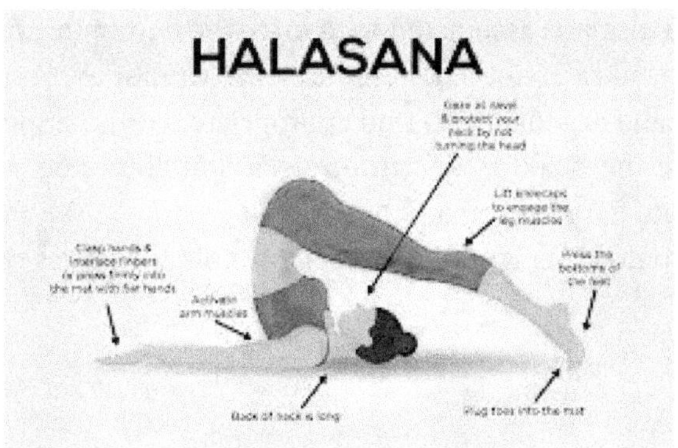

Halasana Fig2

Halasana helps to stretch your spine and even tones the back muscles. It also provides strength to shoulders, arms and legs. Due to practice of Halasana, the muscles and joints become flexible and their mobility enhances.

This asana helps to achieve weight loss since pressure is applied to stomach and belly region.

Who should Avoid this Pose?

People who have weak or injured cervical muscles, weak legs, and weak hamstring muscles or calf muscles should avoid doing this pose. Women during menstruation and pregnancy should also avoid doing this pose. People who are suffering from thyroid or have enlarged liver and spleen also should avoid this yoga pose.

The benefits of Halasana are:

- Helps to improve digestion
- Helps to relieve Back pain and stress
- It helps to heal Thyroid Gland and diabetes
- It is a therapeutic for Leg Cramps. ...
- It helps improve blood circulation
-

Summary

1. The Throat chakra is located at the base of the throat. The color blue is related to it and it is associated with effective communication.
2. When the chakra is not balanced, then we cannot express our thoughts effectively and are unable to find appropriate words to speak.
3. To improve the chakra, we can do neck stretches, and yoga poses like Halasana and Sarvangasana.
4. We can also do affirmations and use blue colored stones or crystals.

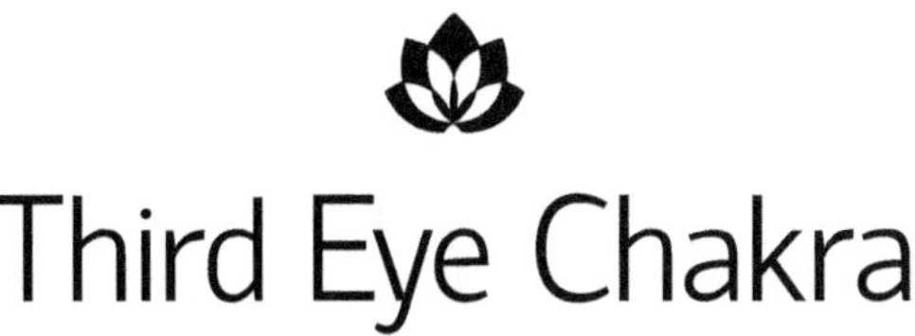

CHAPTER SEVEN

Third Eye Chakra

The other name of this chakra is Ajna chakra. It is associated with light or brightness. It is present in between the two eyebrows and approximately at the center of the forehead. The color of this chakra is indigo.

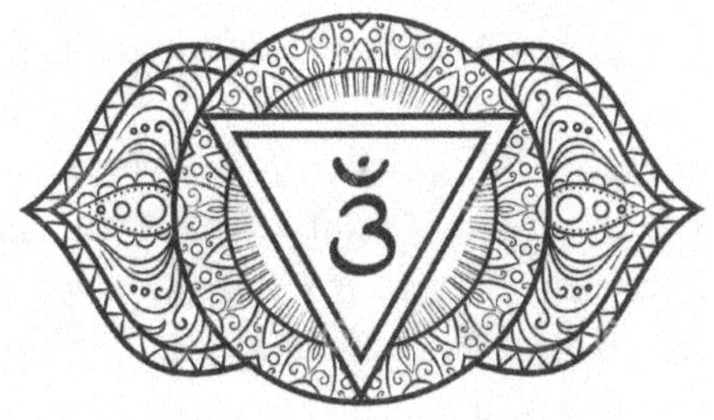

Third Eye chakra Fig 1

This chakra is associated with spiritual communication, awareness, and perception of a person in his life. When this chakra is active, it provides us wisdom and insight, and our spiritual connection with God becomes deeper.

Location	Center of forehead between the two eyebrows
Color	Indigo
Element	Light
Seed Mantra	Om

Third Eye Details

Indigo being the color of wisdom helps bring clarity to all the 5 senses of the body. It helps in energies being transformed from the lower chakras to vibrations of high spiritual value.

Imbalance

When this chakra is blocked or imbalanced, we are disconnected from our true selves and develop a desire for material things. We become impatient and are very much living with the burdens of the past. Our vision is blocked by negative thoughts. In this situation, our intuition is blurred and we become indecisive, confused, depressed, and lose our focus completely. We start doubting ourselves and our decisions and so it becomes difficult to achieve our goals.

Generally, an overactive Ajna chakra is not common since our modern lifestyle dominates our physical reality. There are some circumstances where, because of overactive third eye chakra, psychic activities become predominant and it can lead to hallucinations. The person is completely dissociated from the real world.

Due to imbalances in the Ajna chakra, the neurons of the brain are affected and we might experience problems like

1. Headache or Migraine
2. Eye problems
3. Imbalances in the Endocrine system
4. Insomnia

It can also cause disorders in the pituitary and Pineal gland and even Hypothalamus.

Healing the Chakra

To balance the Ajna chakra, it is important to have patience and a state of awareness. If this chakra is balanced, it improves both the spiritual and physical state of an individual. A person develops strong intuition power as he can listen to the voice of inner wisdom. He can take corrective actions and decisions due to balanced emotions and logic.

If a person has an overactive Ajna Chakra, he must spend more time with nature, so that the overwhelming energies of the mind become calm. Since the person is connected to the earth, it activates the feeling of being grounded to the earth.

Yoga techniques to activate the Ajna Chakra

The opening of the Third Eye chakra helps transform life as it improves inner awareness. Since it is a spiritual practice, the Yoga asanas help in complete focus to activate the energy of the third eye chakra.

Headstand or Shirshasana - This is the best way to activate the third eye chakra. If practiced daily, it helps in the proper functioning of the brain and all other sensory organs connected to the brain. It helps to revitalize all the body systems and also helps in solving problems of menopause.

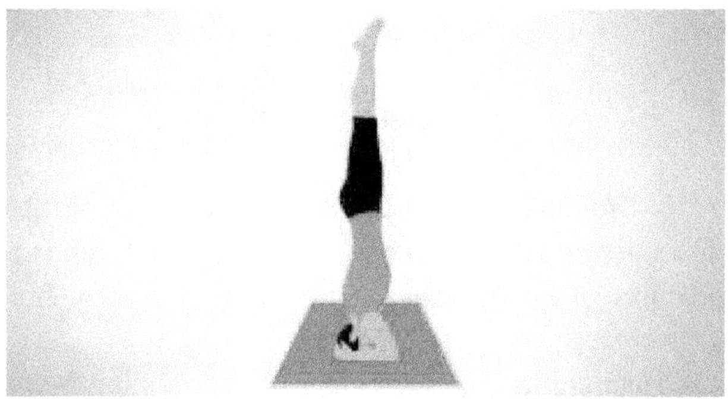

shirshasana Fig1

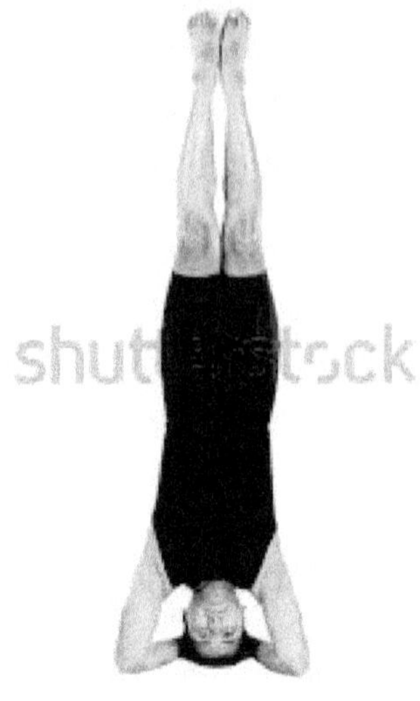

Shirshasana Fig 2

Headstand is also known as the King of asanas. In this, the entire body is inverted as a person has to stand on the top of the head. It is one of the important postures of Hatha Yoga, which is beneficial for both body and mind.

Analysis of Headstand

When a person stands in Shirshasana, the entire body is inverted, at the same time blood pressure is also inverted. The pressure change is experienced in the head, neck, shoulders, veins, arteries, lungs, and legs. This causes the body to work in such a way that it maintains balance in different body systems. It also causes stress and activeness in the upper body parts.

Some people may think that by this pose, blood pressure will increase in the head. But, our body knows how to see that the body and brain carry on their normal functions as they should. If a person is physically well then under the guidance of a Yoga Instructor, he can do this Yoga which will be safe and beneficial. By this pose, the blood pressure in the feet and legs becomes almost zero and in the head increase, and by this various physiological benefits can be seen.

Who should not practice the yoga Headstand?

• Children below the age of 7 years whose skull are not hardened enough should not practice this.

• Pregnant woman should avoid this pose as they might encounter a risk of falling out while doing this pose.

• People suffering from glaucoma, should not do this yoga as it might increase pressure in the eyes.

• Those that have severe headaches and migraine should not opt for this pose.

• People with neck and shoulder injuries also should not perform this till they are healthy.

• People with hypertension and cardiac problems should also avoid this Yoga position.

• Osteoporosis patients should also avoid this.

How to do Headstand?

1. First sit on the knees and measure the ideal distance with the help of elbows. Then bringing your arms under the shoulders keep them to the ground.

2. keeping the elbows there bring the hands closer and interlock the fingers such that the arms form a triangle.

3. Cup the hands and place the back of the head and the other part of the head on the ground.

4. Curling your toes keep your hips to the sky and straighten your knees.

5. Start walking towards your shoulders.

6. Bring the right and left knee towards your chest one by one. This makes the spine straight.

• While inhaling, raise both legs to the sky. Keep your focus at eye level and remain in this pose as long as you feel comfortable and take easy breaths.

Tips to Practice this Yoga

For practicing this Yoga, correct alignment is important else it may lead to injuries. The original name of this pose is Salamba Shirshasana and commonly known as Shirshasana.

1. First it is required to stay in Shashankasana (Child Pose) for 10-15 seconds so that stable blood pressure is maintained in the legs and head before going to Headstand.

2. From the child pose, then place your hands above the head and the elbows should be in line with the shoulders, which gives maximum stability.

3. When placing the head on the ground, remember not to place the crown on the ground, instead place the part of the head that starts from the hairline going to the crown. Standing on the crown is challenging and causes misalignment of the neck.

Breathing to activate Ajna Chakra

For this, sit in a comfortable place with the spine straight. Concentrate on the Third eye location and chant the seed mantra –Om, with full awareness. Continue this for 5 to 15 minutes.

Summary

1. This is also known as Ajna Chakra and is located in the center of the forehead between the two eyebrows.
2. The color is indigo blue and it is associated with light or illumination. It helps us connect with the divine.
3. If the Chakra is imbalanced, then we can feel depressed, we may run after worldly desires and feel disconnected from the divine.
4. To balance this Chakra, we can do Shirshasana, or breathing by concentrating on this chakra and even chanting the beej Mantra OM.

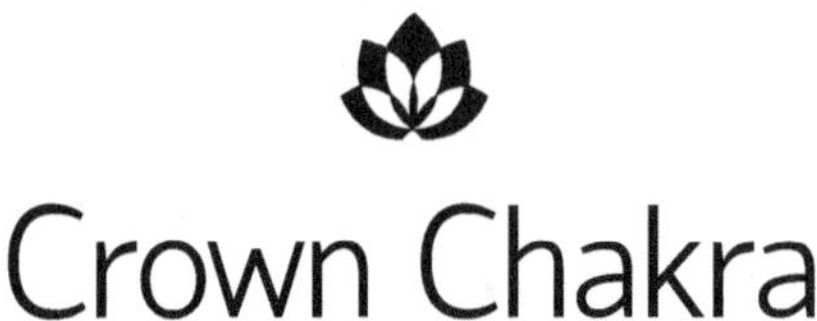

CHAPTER EIGHT

Crown Chakra

The other name of this chakra is the Sahasrara chakra and is located at the top of the head. The color of this chakra is violet. This chakra helps in connecting us to our consciousness, spirit, and self-awareness. It controls our wisdom and unity.

Location	Top of the head
Color	Violet
Element	Spiritual Enlightenment
Seed Mantra	AUM

crown chakra details

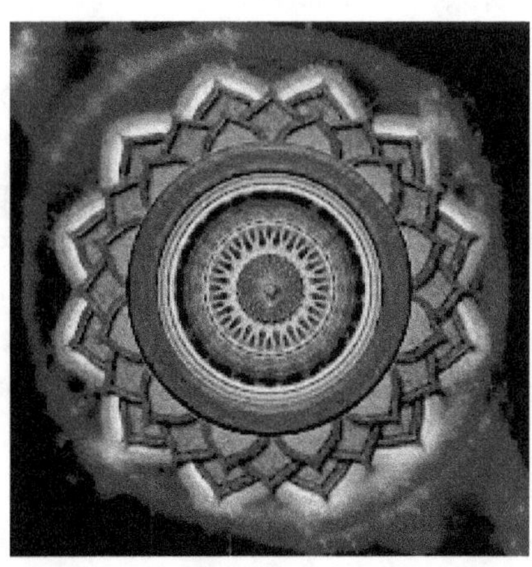

Crown chakra

Since the color is violet, it helps in connecting with spirituality and gives us enlightenment. The glands connected to it are Hypothalamus and Pituitary.

It creates a connection with the supreme self. When the crown chakra is active, it helps in spiritual enlightenment and the flow of universal energy. This is represented by white light. The seed mantra is AUM. This chakra controls brain functions like memory, intelligence, and sharp focus.

Balanced Chakra Characteristics

When the Sahasrara chakra is active, a person gets a positive outlook towards life. The habits and attitude of the person change visibly. Ego does not rule the self and emotions like gratitude, compassion and acceptance become one's true self. In a way, it is a rejection of negative thoughts that can be a cause of unhappiness in life. We experience spiritual understanding and peace when the crown chakra is active. One may experience melancholy, boredom, disillusionment if the crown chakra is unbalanced.

The spiritual essence of violet color

The violet color of this chakra is the color of spirituality. This color has all the qualities of other chakras. It is a unifying color.

The color violet, when activated, helps us to look beyond physical and material values at the spiritual level. It gives us an emotion of letting go of things and brings a great transformation into our perspective. It helps us enjoy the profound change in ourselves.

Signs of a blocked Crown Chakra

We come to know that the Crown Chakra is blocked when we see someone who is too much involved in materialistic things and does not develop a wide way of thinking. He may not accept new ideas, thoughts or even does not want to be open to a new sort of knowledge. When this chakra is imbalanced, a person may be disconnected and does not feel grounded.

When the crown chakra is overactive, then one can notice the following symptoms:

• Pessimism

• Unconcern or indifference

• Spiritual addiction

- Suicidal tendencies
- moved by the knowledge

When the Crown chakra is underactive, then one can notice the following symptoms:

- Confused about what to do in life.
- Lack of inspiration
- Tendency to oversleep

We can see the following physical symptoms when the Crown Chakra is blocked:

- Unable to manage things properly
- Anxiety leading to headaches
- Extreme tiredness

Crown Chakra meditations

Since this seventh chakra helps us in developing spiritual intellect, its energy is supported by all other six chakras. So it is important to work on the six chakras first to activate the Crown chakra.

All meditations are good for opening all the seven chakras. Meditation helps us gain self-awareness and relaxation.

The following are the steps for crown chakra meditation

- Sit comfortably with spine erect and feet resting on the floor
- Place your hands on your knees with palms facing the sky.
- Close your eyes and start inhaling through the nose and exhaling through the mouth.
- While inhaling and exhaling imagine white petals of a lotus outspreading gradually.
- Visualize a bright light surrounding your crown area of the head and gradually spreading throughout your body
- After 5 to 10 minutes open your eyes and sit for a few seconds absorbing that feeling of visualization.

We can also chant the mantra AUM which leads to deep meditation and healing of the chakra.

Yoga asana for activating the Crown Chakra

Some Yoga poses beneficial to awaken the Crown chakra are those in which the forehead touches the ground. They can also be in seated postures.

Here are three yoga asana that can be easily performed to balance the Crown Chakra:

- **Headstand | Shirshasana –**

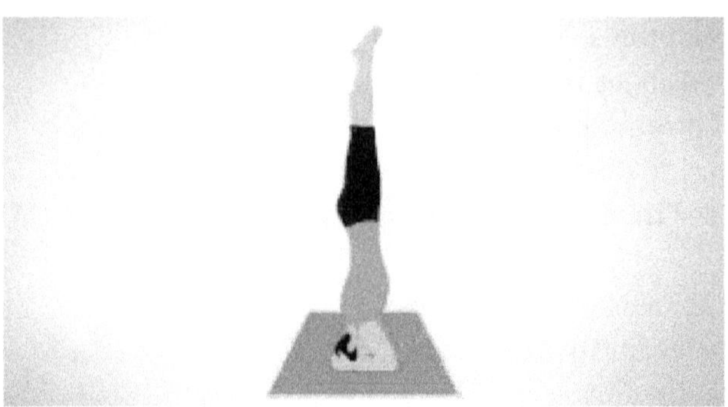

Enter Caption

This Yoga asana is ideal to stimulate energy in the crown chakra. In this posture, the core muscles are engaged and help to provide strength and energy. This posture can be done with five easy breaths. If one practices this posture regularly, it gives clarity of mind.

- **Rabbit Pose | Sasangasana –**

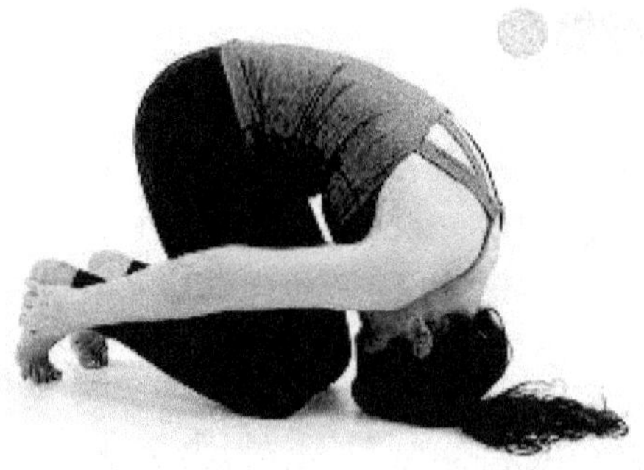

Rabbit pose Fig 1

Rabbit Pose is an excellent way to deeply connect with the Crown Chakra. It helps to relax the head, spine, and shoulders.

- This pose helps in a deep connection with the Crown chakra. It relaxes the head, spine, and shoulders.
- First, kneel down, and then bend forward by bringing the crown of your head towards the floor.
- Move your arms backward and then cup the heels with your hands.
- Without applying pressure on the head, lightly touch the floor.
- After several breaths, release the grip of your hands from the heels and lower your hips towards the heels. Then straighten your spine in a sitting position.

Corpse Pose | Halasana

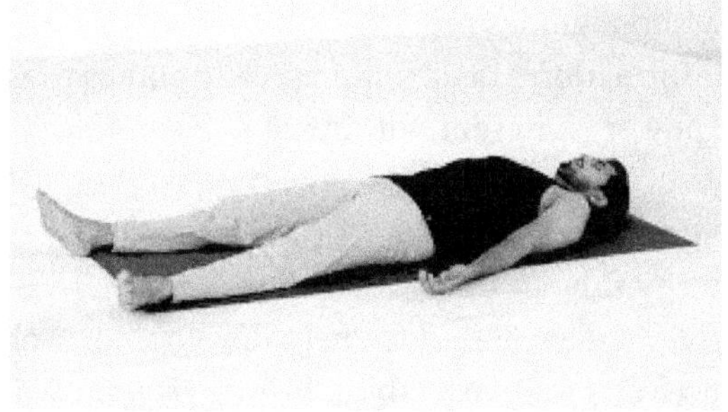

corpse Pose Fig1

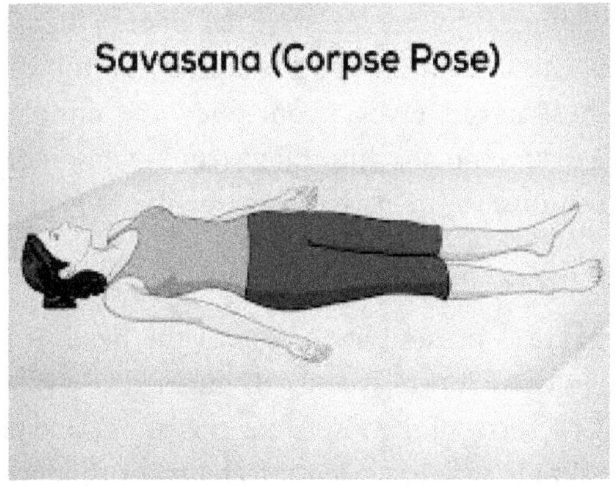

corpse Pose Fig2

This is the most effective yoga asana which helps in practicing detachment. By practicing this, one can learn to let go of desires and expectations. We do not go into too much judgment. By visualizing a white light originating from the crown chakra and moving through the entire length of the spine, as we inhale, we can reap its benefits. As we exhale, we can visualize the same white light rising up to the crown chakra from the spine.

Use Positive affirmations to Open the Crown Chakra

The best technique to balance any chakra is using positive affirmations. These affirmations help individuals gain confidence and faith in themselves without any involvement of Ego. Some affirmations for Crown chakra are

- The higher power guides me
- The inner wisdom guides me
- Whatever information I need automatically comes to me
- The Divine power is present within me
- I am ready to accept new ideas
- This world is my Teacher

Foods for energy flow in the Crown chakra

Various natural, wholesome foods help develop our well-being. Various fresh and organic fruits and vegetables, brown rice, brown bread, and also some broths help to align our chakras. There are violet eggplant and grapes related to crown chakra which is useful. Ginger spices and herbal teas are useful for removing blockages and improving the digestive system.

Conclusion

Each chakra being a source of spiritual energy helps us understand ourselves better. The Crown chakra present at the top of the head helps us feel completeness in ourselves. If our body and mind are balanced and in peace, we can overcome any hindrances and even emotional blockages, which will help us move to the path of spirituality.

Summary

1. The crown chakra is present at the top of the head. It is violet in color and is related to consciousness and self-awareness.
2. To activate this chakra all the lower chakras are also balanced.
3. When this chakra is active, we learn to let go of things and look beyond all physical and material things.
4. When it is blocked then we are unable to manage things, develop anxiety, etc.

5. To open this chakra, we can do Yoga Poses like Shirshasana, Rabbit Pose, or Shavasana.

6. We can do certain positive affirmations and consume foods related to this chakra.

CHAPTER NINE

How to Know the Location of the Chakras

It is important for us to know the location of the chakras with the help of our hands and fingers in our bodies.

Let us see how

1. Place the little finger of your hand on the Manipura chakra or navel.

2. Stretch your hand upwards and see where the tip of the thumb touches, is actually the Heart chakra.

3. Now, in this region, place your little finger again, extend your hand upwards to see where the thumb touches, which is the throat chakra.

4. From the throat chakra, placing your little finger, extend the hand upwards and see where the thumb touches, which is the third eye chakra.

5. Now again, place your little finger on this chakra, extend your hands up and see where your thumb touches, which is the crown chakra.

6. Now again go back to the Manipura and this time place your thumb on it and extend your hands downwards and see where your little finger touches, which is the sacral chakra.

7. Now place your thumbs on the sacral chakra and from there extend your hands downwards and see where the little finger touches, which is the root chakra or muladhara.

Afterward

Though I am a Teacher of computers and English, topics like Yoga, chakras, occult sciences, Law of Attraction attract me very much.

Although I have written various books on the computer Languages I teach, I wanted to write books on the topics that interest me much, so I started reading articles, books, and magazines and finally came up with this topic on the seven chakras.

I have given concise information for each chakra along with the Yogas necessary for each chakra and their seed mantras. I have tried to give relevant information regarding each chakra to the best of my knowledge.

In case of any suggestions and feedback, please contact me on
jashpritma@gmail.com

www.ingramcontent.com/pod-product-compliance
Lightning Source LLC
Chambersburg PA
CBHW061333120726
48001CB00002B/840